# Forensic Psychotherapy



Forensic psychotherapy explores the roots of violent, sexual and antisocial behaviour. It is a relatively recently created discipline that applies psychoanalytic knowledge to the assessment, management and treatment of mentally disordered offenders, forming a bridge between traditional forensic psychiatry – with its focus on diagnosis and risk – and traditional psychotherapy – with its focus on understanding why things happen. As a discipline, forensic psychotherapy seeks to understand the conscious and unconscious motivations that underpin specific offending behaviours. We need to understand not only the detail of the crime, but also the offender as a whole person within his environment, including the criminal justice environment. It aims to understand the perpetrator, the victim and the victim within the perpetrator.

In this collection, leading international experts in forensic psychotherapy explore the different aspects and developments within the field. These include first hand experiences of shaping the emerging discipline within the UK, Europe and the United States; working therapeutically with high-risk offenders in prisons and secure hospitals; exploration of female violence and work with incarcerated mothers and babies; and the latest developments in forensic psychotherapy training. This book will be of interest to professionals and academics working within the fields of forensic mental health, criminal justice, psychiatry, psychology, criminology, and sociology.

This book was originally published as two special issues of *Psychoanalytic Psychotherapy*.

**Jessica Yakeley** is a Consultant Psychiatrist in Forensic Psychotherapy and Director of the Portman Clinic, Tavistock and Portman NHS Foundation Trust, London, UK.

**Gill McGauley** was Professor of Forensic Psychotherapy and Medical Education at St. George's, University of London, UK; and Consultant Forensic Psychotherapist, Central and North West London NHS Foundation Trust.

**To Gill**

# Forensic Psychotherapy

*Edited by*

**Jessica Yakeley and Gill McGauley**

Routledge
Taylor & Francis Group
LONDON AND NEW YORK

First published 2018 by Routledge

2 Park Square, Milton Park, Abingdon, Oxfordshire OX14 4RN
52 Vanderbilt Avenue, New York, NY 10017

*Routledge is an imprint of the Taylor & Francis Group, an informa business*

First issued in paperback 2019



*British Library Cataloguing in Publication Data*
A catalogue record for this book is available from the British Library

ISBN 13: 978-0-415-78953-0 (hbk)
ISBN 13: 978-0-367-22961-0 (pbk)

Typeset in Times New Roman
by RefineCatch Limited, Bungay, Suffolk

# Contents

# Citation Information

The following chapters were originally published in *Psychoanalytic Psychotherapy*, volume 29, issue 3 (September 2015). When citing this material, please use the original page numbering for each article, as follows:

**Chapter 1**
*Forensic psychotherapy*
Estela Welldon
*Psychoanalytic Psychotherapy*, volume 29, issue 3 (September 2015), pp. 211–227

**Chapter 2**
*Female violence and toxic couples*
Anna Motz
*Psychoanalytic Psychotherapy*, volume 29, issue 3 (September 2015), pp. 228–242

**Chapter 3**
*3 Man unlock: out of sight, out of mind – Art psychotherapy with a woman with severe and dangerous personality disorder in prison*
Jessica Collier
*Psychoanalytic Psychotherapy*, volume 29, issue 3 (September 2015), pp. 243–261

**Chapter 4**
*The place of psychoanalytic psychotherapy in the treatment of high-risk personality-disordered offenders*
Celia Taylor
*Psychoanalytic Psychotherapy*, volume 29, issue 3 (September 2015), pp. 262–275

**Chapter 5**

*'This is the pain I feel!' Projection and emotional pain in the nurse–patient relationship with people diagnosed with personality disorders in forensic and specialist personality disorder services: findings from a mixed methods study*
Anne Aiyegbusi and Daniel Kelly
*Psychoanalytic Psychotherapy*, volume 29, issue 3 (September 2015), pp. 276–294

**Chapter 6**

*Safety in numbers: group therapy-based index offence work in secure psychiatric care*
Gwen Adshead
*Psychoanalytic Psychotherapy*, volume 29, issue 3 (September 2015), pp. 295–310

The following chapters were originally published in *Psychoanalytic Psychotherapy*, volume 30, issue 2 (June 2016). When citing this material, please use the original page numbering for each article, as follows:

**Chapter 7**

*Can psychoanalysis help us to understand the causes and prevention of violence?*
James Gilligan
*Psychoanalytic Psychotherapy*, volume 30, issue 2 (June 2016), pp. 125–137

**Chapter 8**

*Forensic follow-up care for outpatients in Germany*
Markus G. Feil
*Psychoanalytic Psychotherapy*, volume 30, issue 2 (June 2016), pp. 138–151

**Chapter 9**

*Creating mother and baby therapy groups in prison: emotional valuation*
Pamela Windham Stewart
*Psychoanalytic Psychotherapy*, volume 30, issue 2 (June 2016), pp. 152–163

**Chapter 10**

*A child's loss becomes a young man's violence*
Carine Minne
*Psychoanalytic Psychotherapy*, volume 30, issue 2 (June 2016), pp. 164–177

**Chapter 11**

*In praise of Dr Leslie Sohn 1919–2013*
Carine Minne
*Psychoanalytic Psychotherapy*, volume 30, issue 2 (June 2016), pp. 178–181

**Chapter 12**

*A fertile matrix: the birth of the Forensic Psychotherapy Society*
Gabriel Kirtchuk, John Gordon, Ronald Doctor and Richard Ingram
*Psychoanalytic Psychotherapy*, volume 30, issue 2 (June 2016), pp. 181–195

# Notes on Contributors

**Gwen Adshead** is a Consultant Forensic Psychiatrist and Psychotherapist at the Department of Forensic Psychiatry, Ravenswood House, Fareham, Hampshire, UK.

**Anne Aiyegbusi** is Deputy Director of Nursing, Specialist and Forensic Services at West London Mental Health NHS Trust, Middlesex, UK.

**Jessica Collier** is an Art Psychotherapist at Offender Care Services, Central and North West London NHS Foundation Trust, London, UK.

**Ronald Doctor** is a Consultant Psychiatrist in Medical and Forensic Psychotherapy at the Psychotherapy Service, West Middlesex Hospital and the Ealing Forensic Psychotherapy Services, West London Mental Health NHS Trust, Isleworth, UK. He is the Training Program Director of the West London Higher Training Scheme in Psychotherapy.

**Markus G. Feil** is the Director of the Psychotherapeutic Outpatient Clinic for Violence and Sexual Offenders, Evangelisches Hilfswerk München gemeinnützige GmbH, Munich, Germany.

**James Gilligan** is a Clinical Professor at the Department of Psychiatry, School of Medicine, New York University, New York, NY, USA.

**John Gordon** is a Consultant Adult Psychotherapist, Psychoanalyst and Group Analyst at the Forensic Psychotherapy Department, West London Mental Health NHS Trust, London, UK.

**Richard Ingram** is a Consultant Psychiatrist at the Centre for Psychotherapy, Belfast Trust, Belfast, UK.

**Daniel Kelly** is Director of Research and RCN Chair of Nursing Research at the School of Healthcare Sciences, College of Biomedical and Life Sciences, Cardiff University, UK.

**Gabriel Kirtchuk** is a Consultant Psychiatrist at the Forensic Psychotherapy Department, West London Mental Health NHS Trust, London, UK.

**Gill McGauley** was Professor of Forensic Psychotherapy and Medical Education at St. George's, University of London, UK; and Consultant Forensic Psychotherapist, Central and North West London NHS Foundation Trust.

**Carine Minne** is a Consultant Psychiatrist in Forensic Psychotherapy at the Portman Clinic, Tavistock and Portman NHS Foundation Trust, London, UK.

**Anna Motz** is a Consultant Clinical and Forensic Psychologist at the Oxford Clinic and Littlemore Mental Health Centre, Oxford, UK. She is the former President of the International Association for Forensic Psychotherapy.

**Celia Taylor** is the Founder of the Millfields Unit, John Howard Centre, East London NHS Foundation Mental Health Trust, London, UK, and a Senior Clinician at the London Pathways Partnership, UK.

**Estela Welldon** is the Founder and Honorary Elected President for Life of the International Association for Forensic Psychotherapy, a Fellow of the Royal College of Psychiatrists, a Senior Member of the British Association for Psychotherapy, a member of the American Group Analysis, of the British Psychoanalytic Council, of the International Association of Group Psychotherapy and of the Confederation of British Psychotherapists.

**Pamela Windham Stewart** is a Psychotherapist at HMP Bronzefield and HMP Holloway, London, UK.

**Jessica Yakeley** is a Consultant Psychiatrist in Forensic Psychotherapy and Director of the Portman Clinic, Tavistock and Portman NHS Foundation Trust, London, UK.

# DEDICATION

## Making minds more secure: Remembering Gill McGauley

Forensic psychiatry and psychotherapy lost a major voice and thinker in July 2016 when Professor Gill McGauley died suddenly and unexpectedly, only three weeks after she had been diagnosed with cancer of the oesophagus. This was a cruel and devastating loss; and especially painful because her family, friends and colleagues in the field of forensic psychotherapy had rejoiced with her in May when she gave her inaugural address as Professor of Medical Education and Forensic Psychotherapy at St George's Hospital, London.

These types of loss are hard to articulate, or make sense of: there is a terrible irony here that Gill herself would be the best person to help us think about it. As many will know, Gill had made a particular study of attachment theory as it applied to forensic psychiatry, and had carried out important research into the childhood histories and attachment representations of violent offenders with severe personality disorders. Together with Luisa Avellan, she helped us to think about how a disorganized attachment system might have devastating effects on the capacity to be pro-social and to mentalise distress in adulthood. She was a member of an active group at Broadmoor Hospital, which sought to explore how her research, and that of Fonagy & Bateman (2008, 2016), could be applied to the development of therapeutic interventions for men and women who were not only high risk offenders, but also suffered mental illness and personality disorder.

Gill was kind and funny and clever; wearing her learning lightly, and also managing to handle with grace and patience the distressing material we work with every day as forensic psychotherapists. She would be the first to say that she was supported in this work by her family's love and care, and also by her time as a patient in psychoanalysis. The psychoanalytic frame of reference helped her maintain that 'third position' that is crucial to forensic work, both in individual work, and at the organizational level. She was a valued member of the reflective practice team at Broadmoor, which tried to support and enable ward staff to care for forensic patients in long stay care; a job which is hard because it is complex, and emotionally laborious.

Gill was my friend and colleague for over 30 years; we trained at medical school together, and in psychiatry in London. We worked together in forensic psychiatry, we both became intrigued by the possibilities of forensic psychotherapy at the same time, trained in the use of the Adult Attachment Interview at the same time, and worked together as consultants in forensic psychotherapy at Broadmoor Hospital for over a decade. We were working together on a book chapter for an international work when she became ill; and it will be painful to see it published without her, as well as this volume that has emerged from the two Special Issues of Forensic Psychotherapy published in *Psychoanalytic Psychotherapy*, for which she was Guest Editor. She would want us to carry on her work, though: to continue to study complex psychopathology to the best of our abilities; to explore therapeutic interventions and their efficacy; and to help develop the careers of young forensic psychotherapists, so that we have more Gill-like minds to help us in the work. Her friends and colleagues will grieve in many ways and at many times in the future, but perhaps especially for the future colleagues who will not have the pleasure of knowing Professor Gill McGauley.

## References

Bateman, A., & Fonagy, P. (2008). Comorbid antisocial and borderline personality disorders: mentalization-based treatment. *Journal of clinical psychology*, *64*(2), 181–194.

Bateman, A., O'Connell, J., Lorenzini, N., Gardner, T., & Fonagy, P. (2016). A randomised controlled trial of mentalization-based treatment versus structured clinical management for patients with comorbid borderline personality disorder and antisocial personality disorder. *BMC psychiatry*, *16*(1), 304.

Gwen Adshead
September 26th 2016

# FOREWORD[1]

## Gill McGauley and Jessica Yakeley

This book, first published as two volumes of a Special Edition of Forensic Psychotherapy in *Psychoanalytic Psychotherapy*, and with Gill McGauley as Guest Editor, provides the reader with a wide ranging selection of papers from prominent forensic psychotherapists in the UK, Germany and the United States, show-casing the contribution of forensic psychotherapy and its applications both to the treatment of offender patients and to the understanding of the dynamics of the patient–professional relationship.

Forensic psychotherapy refers to the application of psychoanalytic principles and treatment in the service of understanding, treating and caring for mentally disordered offenders (Welldon, 1994). Why should we be interested in these men and women that, in the main, we lock away? In England and Wales we live in a society that has the highest rate of imprisonment per head of population in the old European Union (Walmsley, 2003) and 9 out of 10 prisoners have at least one mental disorder but co-morbidity is the norm (Singleton et al, 1997). We also detain considerable numbers of people in secure hospitals or units on Ministry of Justice Restriction Orders. We have suggested elsewhere (Bartlett and McGauley, 2010) that we need to be interested in what happens to those individuals while they are locked away and after they cease to be detained, not just because we are responsible professionals but because how we care for those individuals we deem to have transgressed societal rules may be important markers of our own humanity.

Forensic psychotherapy is intimately concerned with the triangulated and oscillating dynamic between the patient, the psychotherapist and society often represented by the criminal justice system, and Estela Welldon's opening paper eloquently describes this as well as two other triangulations commonly found when working with the forensic patient: the triangulated power dynamics alive in roles such as the 'bully', the 'victim' and the 'bystander' (sometimes intervening as 'rescuer'), drawing on the work Twemlow, and the tripartite cultures of blaming, of concern and of learning. All too often the primitive defence mechanisms of splitting, projection and projective identification become mobilized both in violence and in the commonly evoked blaming and retaliatory responses to violence or sexual abuse. Welldon encourages us to raise society's awareness of these powerful unconscious processes; salient in the light of the violent, terrorising and sectarianism attacks that we human beings perpetrate on each other. Welldon's paper contains many more rich ideas as she describes the history of

[1] This foreword is an adapted version of the two editorials published in the respective Special Issues of Forensic Psychotherapy.

forensic psychotherapy and, of course, she is a part of that history having pioneered the development of forensic psychotherapy nationally and internationally over the last four decades and founded the International Association of Forensic Psychotherapy in 1991. Welldon describes, with apposite clinical examples, the particular theoretical and practical considerations that are needed when working with forensic patients; for example the unconscious meaning of the offence; the nature of the transference and countertransference and the containing role of the institution, its staff and its structures. Welldon's paper closes with her own theoretical and clinical contribution to the field in her discussion of the different aims of male and female perversions. In brief her differentiation is that, in men, the act is aimed at an outside part-object, whereas in women it is usually aimed against themselves, either against their bodies or against objects which they see as their own creations, that is, their babies. In both cases, bodies and babies are treated as part-objects.

The task of forensic psychotherapy may be distilled into one overarching aim: to increase the person's pro-social capacity and to decrease risk to others; although the latter outcome would follow if the first part of the aim was achieved. Many of the papers in this book provide compelling clinical accounts of individual, group and art psychotherapy with men and women who have offended, often violently, towards men, women and children to whom they have an attachment relationship as partners, parents or as the children of those they have attacked. The overarching theoretical model that the authors most often draw upon, either explicitly or implicitly, is that of attachment theory and the developmental capacities that arise from it, such as mentalization. Mentalization theory integrates psychoanalytic thinking with attachment theory and research and refers to the wish and the capacity to understand interpersonal behaviour in terms of mental states, of our self and of others.

Gwen Adshead describes how psychodynamic group work is a pro-socialising process drawing from her experience of facilitating a long-term group for men detained in a high secure hospital who have killed when mentally ill; a group of individuals who would traditionally be excluded from psychodynamic work. Adshead proposes that, as group members, these men develop non-malevolent attachment relationships through which they can explore their responsibility for their offences. By allowing unconscious agency to become more conscious, in other words through fostering the capacity to mentalize aspects of their own minds and the minds of others in the presence of the group members, these men can begin a process of recovery and their risk to others can reduce. Adshead and her colleagues have paid detailed attention to subtle changes in their patients' narratives over time. She marshals a persuasive empirical and theoretical argument that these increases in narrative coherence may well be proxy markers of an increases in mentalization.

Central to Anna Motz's paper on female violence is the notion that the dual role of perpetrator and victim can coexist in the same person and that either of these internal aspects may gain the ascendancy across different stages of the lifespan. Motz provides a transgenerational perspective on the sequelae of early abuse within the context of attachment relationships describing how, for some women, the effects of early perverse attachment experiences can be unconsciously recreated in the woman's adult life towards her partner and/or her children. She cautions that it is essential to keep in mind that women too can be violent perpetrators within the domestically violent couple. Drawing on Welldon's work on maternal perversion Motz describes her patient's cruelty towards her daughter in a repetition of the patient's experiences of her own early abuse. Motz's descriptions of treatment illustrate how we can feel the pull of projective processes attempting to counter-transferentially nudge us into enacting the role of either the victim or aggressor. At these moments we, as psychotherapists, need to sustain our capacity to mentalize while remaining with our patients in the eye of the psychic storm.

Motz proposes that the 'toxic couple', where it is the relationship rather than the individuals which is toxic, arises from the interaction of two disturbed attachment systems. Motz's clinical accounts chart the developmental burden of poor early attachment; namely a fragile capacity to mentalize. It is precisely when the attachment system is activated, either in the toxic coupling of partner or parental attachments, that this already compromised capacity to mentalize is most vulnerable. When mentalization fractures, violence erupts. Motz's clinical examples underline the fact that mentalization is a function of the social mind: to fully mentalize you need another or to envision the mind of another.

So from group work in a high secure hospital, through consideration of couple dynamics in community settings we move to Jessica Collier's paper which focusses on individual art psychotherapy within the challenging environment of a women's prison. Forensic art psychotherapists are often the people that offer treatment to patients who evoke feelings of despondency or impotence in clinicians, psychotherapists and other professionals. Collier's paper describes how art psychotherapy helped contain the trauma and violent acting out of an imprisoned woman whose affective dysregulation and capacity for physical violence meant that she could not make contact with another human being unless three others were on hand to potentially restrain her. Collier's wide ranging paper covers aspects such as the necessity for us to carefully monitor our countertransference when working with forensic patients as well as institutional and staff responses which may unwittingly stimulate unconscious re-enactments of abuse and trauma from the patient's past or from the trauma of committing the violent act. However, the key mechanism Collier describes is how, through the therapeutic relationship and the making of images, the patient became more able to introject the split off and projected violent aspects of herself. Mankind has always sought a visual language for narrative and images contain meaning which can provide patients with a narrative through which to express their feelings and see them contained. One way of conceptualizing this process, through the lens of mentalization, is that art psychotherapy helps make the implicit explicit in a way that can be tolerable for highly disturbed minds. In other words, if the individual has a fragile capacity to mentalize then thinking about being a victim of the violence of others or of perpetrating violence cannot be sustained. Images can simultaneously occupy a mental position of being part of 'me' and 'not part of me'; a product of my mind and an externally projected aspect of my experience that I can regulate my distance from. As Collier says, these expressions of a patient's internal world can be put away, kept safe and brought out again when the patient can mentalize. Moreover, as well as providing the patient with this regulatory mechanism the process of art therapy may well strengthen the patient's capacity to mentalize.

Collier and Motz describe their work with patients who have a diagnosis of personality disorder. The next two papers focus on this patient group. Celia Taylor describes how the treatment model at Millfield's Unit, one of the original medium secure services for high-risk personality-disordered offenders, has incorporated a psychoanalytic approach into the overarching therapeutic community (TC) model. This analytic approach has helped to engage men who find it difficult to allow themselves to be helped and has guided staff in their responses to their patients and in managing the risk these men pose to themselves and others. Not only do TCs aim to establish a culture of enquiry that fosters attachment by providing a secure base but the TC model puts mentalization at its core. TCs provide a socialising environment where there are opportunities for aggressive, denigrating or paranoid styles of relating, borne out of early adversity, to be reformulated and reworked within and between individuals. Sadly, Taylor's poignant description of the early life of one of her patients, who killed his parent, illustrate how the prodrome of the index offence can begin years earlier and is rooted in a cruel attachment relationship where the child is treated no better than the family dog. This dehumanization not only wrecks the child's capacity to form secure attachments but damages the development of mentalization. Consequentially trauma cannot be worked through; affect is easily dysregulated and becomes overwhelming; mentalization breaks down and violence erupts as in the case of this patient when he beat his father to death.

Taylor and Aiyegbusi's papers bring an additional perspective, which is crucially important for the survival of forensic psychotherapy and its application, namely that of researching and evaluating the impact of the treatment we provide. Taylor's unit used a quantitative approach with clinician- and patient-rated measures of violent risk and psychiatric symptomatology respectively. Early results showed a decrease in symptomatology but were not so conclusive for risk. Anne Aiyegbusi's paper reports a mixed methods research study which focussed on the nurse–patient relationship in offenders with a diagnosis of personality disorder in one of the Dangerous and Severe Personality Disorder (DSPD) Units, a Women's Enhanced Medium Secure Unit and a TC. The author describes a carefully thought through qualitative methodology designed to examine both the nurses' and the patients' experience of the nurse–patient relationship. The main theme reported in the paper is 'Pain: Processing or Passing on?' In the context of the study this referred to whether and how the nurses contained the patients' projections and challenging behaviours. One interesting finding was that the nurses' therapeutic response appeared to be determined by their prior clinical training which was influenced by the model of care in the services in which they had worked. Nurses who were able to think about (mentalize) the meaning behind their patients' behaviour had received some training in psychodynamic nursing theory and practice and had worked in services where psychodynamic approaches were valued. Aiyegbusi concludes that significant investment in psychodynamic training and supervision is needed for nurses if they are to understand their work in terms of interpersonal processes rather than perceiving themselves as "legitimised emotional punch bags". The national training for working with people with personality disorder, the Knowledge and Understanding Framework (KUF), commissioned by the Department of Health and Ministry of Justice was a welcome development but may not be the most effective model to achieve what Aiyegbusi proposes is needed. The clinical question flowing from Aiyegbusi's work is how does one change the practice of individuals and teams? A model which trains individuals, largely outside of their work context, may not achieve the desired impact on practice through the transfer of skills. An alternative is to get teams to mentalize using a whole team approach such as AMBIT. This mentalization based approach was developed at the Anna Freud Centre in London for teams working with young people with severe needs who are difficult to engage and provides tools for putting mentalization to use in teams in general. It is a whole team approach and facilitates team practice and process by supporting mentalization within teams, between teams and within networks and, as such, may have much to offer us in our therapeutic work.

The next paper interrogates the psychoanalytic foundation of forensic psychotherapy. How can Freud's ideas, originating in his discoveries of treating hysterical women in late nineteenth and early twentieth century Vienna, be applied to the forensic world of murderers and rapists? How can psychoanalysis, which traditionally considers antisocial and violent behaviour as serious contradictions for psychoanalytic treatment, be adapted to the therapeutic needs of offenders? James Gilligan, one of the foremost contemporary psychoanalytic thinkers on violence, proposes that psychoanalysis offers the most powerful cognitive and emotional understanding of the workings of the human psyche than any other method, shifting the philosophical and moral question "How should I live and what should I do?" to the scientific question "How can I live?" i.e. "What processes maintain life, and which forces lead to damage and death?" He asserts that these questions can be empirically examined and tested by applying psychoanalytic theories and methods to the study of human behaviours, including those of extreme violence.

Gilligan relates his own personal and professional journey, starting as a recent graduate from Harvard Medical School taking a job as a prison psychiatrist to support his young family, where he discovered to his surprise that working with convicted criminals and murderers, who had been deemed untreatable sociopaths deserving only punishment and control, was one of the most emotionally moving experiences of his career to date. In this and his subsequent work in the

Massachusetts prison system, where he eventually became the director of mental health services, he discovered that far from being amoral, as was widely believed, murderers and rapists were preoccupied with fundamental questions of morality. Through his work with high-security inmates, he found that their early experiences of being rejected, ostracised, abused or made to feel as if they did not exist, predisposed them as adults to be sensitised to feeling bullied, ignored or "disrespected", leading to unbearable feelings of shame and humiliation which need to be defended against by violent means. Gilligan proposes that certain preconditions increase the likelihood that shame will cause violence: first, that overwhelming shame has obliterated in these men their sense of existence by killing their soul, so that mutilating themselves and others is enacted to make them feel alive; second, because shame also kills the emotion of self-love or pride which mitigates harm to others; third, their lack of education and work that would normally raise self-esteem; and finally, what he calls their 'male role belief system' in which being a man means being superior to others, a status that has to be achieved and maintained through violence.

Gilligan incorporated these ideas into developing and researching a pioneering violence prevention programme in the jails of San Francisco, immersing violent offenders in an intensive therapeutic and educational programme, including group therapy. This programme was awarded a major national prize from the Kennedy School of Government at Harvard for "innovations in American governance," in a competition with some 800 innovative programs from around the country.

Gilligan's monumental work represents an oasis of optimism in the therapeutic desert of American forensic psychiatry, which still tends to be more concerned with conducting forensic medico-legal evaluations than treating offenders. The situation in Germany, however, thanks to recent legislation, has created more fertile soil for the growth of forensic psychotherapy in all of its federal states. Markus Feil, a psychoanalyst, psychiatrist and head of a forensic psychotherapy outpatient clinic in Munich, documents how changes in the German Criminal Code in 2007 spurred the creation of new forensic outpatient clinics to provide follow-up care for criminal and sex offenders released from prison or secure detention under conditions imposed by the court. Acknowledging that this initiative is a positive approach, Feil nevertheless urges us to retain a cautious and discerning attitude in their appraisal. He rightly highlights some of the tensions and questions inherent in forensic psychotherapy: Is the primary aim of treating offenders to reduce risk or improve health? Can psychotherapy have any genuine effect if it is mandatory as part of a treatment order imposed by the courts? When is the therapist obliged to break the patient's confidentiality to disclose information regarding risk? In his thoughtful article, Feil illustrates how these dilemmas may be enacted in the transference and countertransference where therapists may feel pushed into punitive or monitoring, rather than therapeutic, roles and the therapeutic relationship may become a repetition of the offender's earlier disturbed interpersonal relationships. Feil recommends that, in the multidisciplinary treatment of offenders, the advisory role should be separate from the therapeutic, allowing the therapist to best protect the therapeutic space. The provision of on-going supervision and reflective practice for both the individual therapist and the team is also essential.

The next two papers by Pamela Stewart and Carine Minne illustrate some of the various types of forensic psychotherapy – psychoanalytically-informed group therapy for mothers and infants, and individual psychoanalytic psychotherapy for high-risk personality-disordered offenders – being delivered in the UK Criminal Justice System and the National Health System respectively. These two government organisations, with their different purposes (i.e. protection of the public versus improving the health of patients), governance and professional standards, are increasingly working together in initiatives such as the National Offender Personality Disorder (OPD) Pathway Strategy (Joseph & Benefield, 2012), a government programme which has commissioned services and increased the availability of treatments for offenders with personality disorder as well as increasing the knowledge and skills of the workforce managing this challenging group. Although the inception of both Stewart's and Minne's work predate the OPD Pathway, both may be seen as examples of clinical practice which support one of the underlying principles of the strategy in their developmental understanding of the offender within an attachment framework.

Stewart describes her pioneering work with pregnant mothers, and mothers and their babies, in two UK prisons; HMP and YOI Holloway, until recently the largest women's prison, and HMP and YOI Bronzefield, now the largest female prison. She reminds us that the welfare of female offenders within the Criminal Justice System has been relatively neglected despite these women being at high-risk of depression, self-harm and other mental health problems, and that therapeutic service provision is limited.

Stewart underscores two basic principles of forensic psychotherapy, as put forward by Adrian West (1996), that guide her work. The first is that the crime, or "index offence" is considered as a symptom, or a communication with meaning, that the forensic psychotherapist must keep in mind in a non-persecutory, but also non-collusive way. This may involve a struggle for the therapist between the urge to normalise the experience of being with mothers who appear to be tenderly looking after and breast-feeding their babies, and the recognition, without excessive anxiety or condemnation, of their capacity for dangerousness and destruction, enacted in their serious offences. Managing this tension may be facilitated by West's second basic principle of forensic psychotherapy, namely, not to work in isolation but to join with colleagues to support the therapy. Here the therapist must achieve a balance between protecting a certain confidentiality of the group whilst maintaining close relationships with prison staff, who, she rightly reminds us, are with the prisoners all the time, and hence bear the brunt of their disturbance, whilst the forensic psychotherapist has the luxury of coming to the wing for short periods of time at her discretion.

Stewart also highlights how the prison system mirrors and repeats the early disrupted attachments of the woman's early life, with sentences served far from home, sudden prison transfers, or changes in key prison staff, all of which may interrupt therapeutic continuity. Although this is something that the OPD Pathway is trying to address, particularly with new dedicated services for female offenders, Stewart's pre-existing work with these women demonstrates the extent of the practical and emotional challenges faced by individual professionals and the organization as a whole. The task of fostering the mother's capacity to feel "curiosity about the baby" captures the essence of forensic psychotherapeutic work. This entails helping the mothers to discover both their babies' minds and their own minds, and how their rigid thought patterns and lack of curiosity – in other words an impoverished capacity to mentalize – indicate how little emotional validation these women received from their own caregivers in infancy and childhood, and therefore how little emotional validation they may have to draw on as mothers for their babies; a necessary prerequisite to break the patterns of transgenerational abuse that so often form part of the family history of these women.

The cultivation of curiosity and awareness in the offender's mind is a crucial task in the forensic psychotherapeutic endeavour detailed in Carine Minne's paper. She describes her long-term treatment of two patients whom she saw for twice-weekly psychoanalytic psychotherapy in a high secure hospital. She highlights that traumatic losses that so many of these detained patients have experienced in their childhoods and caused breakdowns in adolescence in the form of violent enactments, are in fact preceded by, often unnoticed, breakdowns in infancy, due to the loss or non-existence of a reliable caring primary object to help them negotiate normal development and psychological maturation. Minne's ideas have been shaped by her late colleague and mentor, the psychiatrist, forensic psychotherapist and psychoanalyst Leslie Sohn. Sohn's unique and inspiring work on understanding the violent behaviour of mentally disordered offenders has influenced subsequent generations of forensic psychotherapists, including the authors of this editorial, who, like Minne, were fortunate enough to benefit from his clinical supervision. Minne has written a deeply moving and personal tribute to Sohn, which we are delighted to include in this volume.

Minne proposes that these patients are traumatized three-fold: firstly, by their terrible background histories of losses and abuse, secondly by the offences they committed, and thirdly, by their gradual discovery, during treatment, that they are mentally ill. This conceptualization of their mental disorder reflects another basic tenet of forensic psychotherapy: that every perpetrator has also been a victim, and that their offending may be an, albeit pathological, attempt to reverse the previous losses and traumas inflicted on them.

In the light of these multiple traumas experienced by the patient, Minne proposes that therapy can lead to the development of a post-traumatic stress-type of disorder, caused by increased awareness and understanding, which should be seen as a positive prognostic indicator. She describes the delicate and complex task that the therapist has to negotiate is how to introduce the patient to the unconscious contents of his mind, without either patient or therapist feeling assaulted and overwhelmed by these contents which could lead to states of unbearable anxiety, psychosis or suicidal despair. This requires careful timing and monitoring of therapeutic interventions, constantly gauging how the patient's awareness of his mind is developing and how he is using this awareness, being alert to the manifestation of negative therapeutic responses. Demonstrating the multi-faceted nature of such complicated work, as well as enlisting the support of the multi-professional team in providing a safe and contained setting, Minne also recommends the judicial use of anti-psychotic medication which can sedate the more intense psychotic anxieties of the patient so that psychoanalytic therapy may progress.

These case examples also illustrate how Minne has pioneered the long-term treatment of patients through different levels of security, seeing patients initially in a high secure setting, and continuing their therapy as they progress through medium security until they can be seen as out-patients in the community. Obviously such long-term work requires not only committed and experienced clinicians, but also the understanding and support of the commissioners who fund such treatment, which, in the current economically constrained climate, is becoming increasingly rare.

The final article, by Gabriel Kirtchuk, John Gordon, Ronald Doctor and Richard Ingram, addresses the training of forensic psychotherapists. Kirtchuk, amongst others, was instrumental in negotiating with the Department of Health in the late 1990s the development of dual training posts throughout the UK in forensic psychotherapy where doctors in higher psychiatric training could train in both psychoanalytic psychotherapy and forensic psychiatry. This development followed the Fallon Inquiry into the Personality Disorder Unit at Ashworth Special Hospital where serious and pervasive boundary violations involving patients and staff had occurred. These training posts are now well established and highly sought after by interested psychiatry trainees. However, until recently, this dual training was the only formalized and accredited training pathway to becoming a registered forensic psychotherapist, which was limited to members of the medical profession. To enable people from other professional disciplines such as nursing, social work, psychology and probation to qualify as psychodynamic forensic psychotherapists, new training opportunities were needed. Kirtchuk and colleagues have lead a step-wise multi-professional approach encompassing an escalator model of training with valid and registrable stages of experience. First they developed a two-year MSc in Psychotherapeutic Approaches in Mental Health, building on their long experience of using basic psychoanalytic concepts to train a wide range of multidisciplinary professionals. This MSc is a collaboration between the Forensic Psychotherapy Training Department at West London Mental Health NHS Trust and New Buckinghamshire University and applies a psychoanalytic perspective for multidisciplinary professionals working in general and forensic psychiatric hospitals, community mental health and associated services to understand the individual, group and organisational dynamics which permeate their work. A satellite of the MSc was developed five years ago in Northern Ireland.

More recently, graduates of the MSc, who are qualified as Psychodynamic Practitioners approved by the British Psychoanalytic Council (BPC), may progress to a Post MSc Training leading to a further qualification as a Forensic Psychodynamic Therapist with a new Member Institution of the British Psychoanalytic Council (BPC) – the Forensic Psychotherapy Society (FPS) – and through this registration with the Forensic Psychodynamic Section of the BPC. This further training forms an integrated part of the trainee's core clinical profession and includes academic teaching, participation in experiential groups, supervised therapy of two individual cases and the requirement of personal therapy for the trainee. The FPS provides both a framework for a national, multidisciplinary professional training in psychodynamic forensic psychotherapy as well as being an active post-qualification organisation supporting CPD and other forms of professional development.

We believe that this book is testimony to how a psychoanalytic approach can be of profound importance in contributing to the therapeutic understanding of offenders and forensic patients, as well ensuring optimal training and containment for the professionals and institutions involved in their care. Forensic psychotherapy is comprised of uneasy coalitions between disciplines and paradigms with diverse and sometimes opposing principles – therapeutics and the law, forensic psychiatry and psychoanalysis, moral ethics and scientific empiricism. However, its distinct identity arises from its efforts to maintain a dialectic between the tensions and conflicts existing at its core, from which creativity and innovation may emerge. The authors in this volume succeed in illustrating how these dilemmas are explored and addressed in different political, sociological and cultural contexts, and in thoughtfully discussing the interplay of both the internal world and the social world to the development of psychopathology and violent acting out that characterises the lives of our patients.

## References

Bartlett A., & McGauley G. A. (2010). In A. Bartlett & G. McGauley (Eds.), *Forensic Mental Health; Concepts, Systems and Practice* (pp. xiii–xv). Oxford: Oxford University Press.

Joseph, N., & Benefield, N. (2012). A joint offender personality disorder pathway strategy: An outline summary. *Criminal Behaviour & Mental Health, 22*, 210–217.

Singleton, N., Meltzer, H., & Gatward, R. (1997). *Psychiatric Morbidity among Prisoners in England and Wales*. Office for National Statistics. TSO (The Stationary Office).

Walmsley, R. (2003). *World Prison Population List (fourth edition)* Findings 188 www.rds.homeoffice.gov.uk/rds/pdfs2/r188.pdf

West, A. (1996). The risks of burnout. In C. Cordess & M. Cox (Eds.), *Forensic Psychotherapy: Crime, Psychodynamics and the Offender Patient, Volume II: Mainly Practice* (pp. 229–240). London: Jessica Kingsley.

# Forensic psychotherapy

Estela Welldon

*Independent Practitioner, London, UK*

## Introduction

This edition of the journal looks at the contribution specialist forensic psychotherapy can make to the rigorous disciplines of forensic psychiatry and the law, as well as helping general psychotherapists who encounter forensic issues. As Bluglass (1990, p. 7) put it 'The role of the forensic psychiatrist in confronting and trying to reconcile the differences between the interests of the law and those of psychiatry is a crucial and important one'.

Forensic psychotherapy can help. It is a bridge between traditional forensic psychiatry with a major focus on diagnosis and risk, and traditional psychotherapy with a focus on understanding why things happen. Williams (1991) described the difficulties encountered in the successful bridging of both disciplines. According to Harding (1992), there is an inevitable, and indeed necessary, conflict of values between the forensic psychiatry and criminal justice systems. Evaluations should ideally be conducted independently, according to criteria that correspond to health-based values (Reed Report, 1992).

Forensic psychotherapy seeks to understand the unconscious motivations that underpin specific offending behaviours. We need to understand not only the detail of the crime, but about the individual as a whole person within his environment (including the criminal justice environment). The criminal action is the central fact. Unfortunately, some psychotherapeutic approaches can seem to be a 'soft' option, justifying and rationalizing behaviour to provide 'false understanding'. Our forensic patients use similar mechanisms to conceal their 'real selves' resulting in encapsulation of the offending behaviour and keeping it hidden or minimized. An effective collusion between society and offenders is at work. The criminal action always appears understandable as an action against society, yet at the same time, it is unconsciously a self-destructive act, with harmful effects for the offender also. This aspect of criminality associated with unconscious guilt has been examined by Freud (1915), Glover (1960) and Tuovinen (1973), among others.

Sometimes the criminal behaviour can become explosive, violent and uncontrollable with profound consequences. It can be the equivalent of a neurotic symptom, a sign of personality disorder or of simple criminality (or maybe all three). Pfäfflin (1992) described how the symptom can even be a constructive and healthy reaction. He adds that it is 'conservative', meaning that the patient needs it and keeps it until it can be properly understood and then he can give it up. We must remember the axiom of the paediatrician and psychoanalyst Dr. Donald Winnicott: 'The antisocial tendency (in adolescence) implies hope and it is characterised by an element in it which compels the environment to be important' (1956).

A psychotherapeutic approach does not seek to condone the crime or to excuse the criminal. On the contrary, the object is to help the offender to acknowledge responsibility for his/her acts and thereby helps to protect the offender and society from the perpetration of further crimes (Welldon, 1988). Taking responsibility and understanding what you did, and why, is more than simply saying you regret it: getting there takes hard work from both patient and therapist(s).

At times, the criminal act is the expression of more severe psychopathology; it is secretive, completely encapsulated and split from the rest of the patient's personality, which acts as a defence against a psychotic illness (Hopper, 1991). On the other hand, it can be a calculated act associated with professional, careerist criminality. The forensic psychotherapist can help to clarify these difficult diagnostic issues.

The form of psychotherapy involved in forensic work is different from other forms precisely because society is, willy-nilly, involved. Forensic psychotherapy has gone beyond the special relationship between patient and psychotherapist. It is a triangular situation – patient, psychotherapist and society. This is the first of at least three different triangular situations found in working with the forensic patient.

The second is the existence of the triangular process or power dynamics in social roles such as the 'bully', the 'victim' and the 'bystander' (sometimes intervening as 'rescuer') well described by Twemlow, Sacco, and Williams (1996). A bully repeatedly uses force, either physical or non-physical to shame, humiliate and dominate a victim. Thus a victim is the target for the bully's force and can become depressed, hopeless and enraged at the mockery. The bystander is the audience for the bully–victim drama. These are dialectically determined roles, not people, and can switch around very rapidly. The bystander role is an important and often unrecognised part of the problem. Court appearances and psychotherapy assessments can become part of this dynamic.

The third triangular situation is that of three different 'cultures': of blaming, of concern and of learning. These terms came to mind when I was invited to give the Oxford Brookes University Fellows Lecture in 2004, From the Court to the Couch, and I used them later in my book, *Playing with Dynamite* (Welldon, 2011, p. 142). The culture of blaming is left to the lay public and society at large. The titillating front pages of tabloid newspapers make it very difficult, if not impossible, to understand the inner world of those who offend or the motivations for their crimes. The common blaming and retaliatory responses to violence or sexual abuse are characterised by splitting and projective identification mechanisms (Klein, 1946) that see people as 'good' or 'bad' in a black or white way. 'Good' people need to safeguard their own goodness by locating badness in others. It is essential that we educate the public about these unconscious attitudes that people display, such as in Knox's (2014) recent article, 'The blame and shame society', but perhaps more importantly and topically, it is heartening to see that these concepts are being used more widely in journalism and in popular non-fiction literature, such as Ronson (2015) *So You've Been Publically Shamed.*

Unfortunately, the culture of concern is almost always left to clinicians, social workers and the judiciary. There is a prejudice among some clinicians that judges are not ready to listen about unconscious motivations and what they would perceive as manoeuvring legal processes to diminish the guilt of the accused. On the contrary I have found that many are open and ready to learn and feel better prepared to face their own role. I always felt that they would be only too willing to listen to clinicians and learn from their own experience. This was confirmed in 1991 when, at an annual meeting of the Advisory Group to the Diploma Course, I put forward a proposal for a 'Judges' residential weekend' that would provide judges with a unique opportunity to learn and understand about unconscious motivations of offenders. To my delight, this was taken seriously and action was immediately taken by Tony Lloyd, now Baron Lloyd of Berwick, and a residential weekend was made possible in Windsor in 1991. Later on Matthew Thorpe, now The Rt. Hon Lord Justice Matthew Thorpe, another member of the Advisory Group, followed suit as a family judge and began to convene a series of weekends for the family justice system with the same format, involving Portman Clinic staff. Forensic psychotherapists have to work to influence this broader system.

Altshul (2013, p. 48), in reviewing a paper on forensic psychotherapy by Yakeley and Adshead (2013), described his reservations about the applicability of psychodynamic principles to judicial and legal processes, but goes on to say 'They describe a humane, sophisticated, and civilised position, and they describe it in a thoughtful and scholarly manner. A large part of me hopes they can prove me wrong'. According to Kapoor and Williams (2012, p. 460) 'We simply believe that thinking through the possible unconscious forces at play in a forensic case adds a layer of richness that would otherwise be lost'.

Thinking and listening and learning are needed to acknowledge and understand these perspectives. We need to promote discussion about such issues in a broad arena, the general public, the politicians, the media and other academic disciplines. Perhaps especially, we need to work better with non-governmental organisations (NGOs) who work with offenders and victims – and with these individuals themselves, in a broader context than the clearly defined clinical setting. We should support relevant academic work. This is the learning culture.

Society instinctively views sexual offenders and their victims in distinct and reflex ways. Whereas the treatment of victims is encouraged and everyone is concerned about their welfare, the same does not apply to perpetrators, and lip service may be paid to the fact that victims could easily become perpetrators. 'Splitting' is in full operation. Linked to this I have challenged the stereotype that women tend to be seen as victims and men as perpetrators, especially in instances of sexual abuse. The difficulties in acknowledging a woman's abusing power in motherhood ('they don't do those awful things') may be the result of massive denial, as a way of dealing with this unpalatable truth (Welldon, 1988). Until recently a lack of legislation on female perversion reflected society's total denial of it. The woman is thereby seen as a part-object, or just a receptacle of men's perverse designs. The apparent idealisation of mothers prevalent in society contains a denigrating counterpart. Following on from my work, this theme has been further reviewed and researched by Motz (2009, 2014, 2014) in her psychoanalytic explorations of the nature of female violence, and by Minne (2011) in her clinical work with psychotic women who have killed their children. Many others have described their psychotherapeutic work with both men and women within the prison and maximum-security units (see Aiyegbusi & Kelly, 2012).

Forensic psychotherapy may appear to be a narrow field yet has been able to push boundaries in order to work with offender patients (sometimes in secure settings). Boundaries have been further extended to offer treatment to groups of people not previously seen as suitable for psychotherapy, such as people who were previously referred to as mentally handicapped, later as having learning disabilities and presently as having intellectual disabilities. In the UK, Sinason has pioneered the application of psychodynamic psychotherapy in the treatment of patients affected with intellectual disabilities (Sinason, 2010) and Curen has also written extensively about their psychodynamic work with children and adults with intellectual disabilities (Curen & Sinason, 2010). More recently Corbett (2014) has described a carefully designed specific treatment along psychodynamic lines for children and adults who show offending behaviour, including inappropriate sexual activity. Others, such as Tilman, have described therapeutic work with other marginalised groups within society, such as migrants.

When we began to work with the concept of forensic psychotherapy, we were accused of diluting psychoanalysis and 'losing its preciousness'. But now the modifications from psychoanalysis necessary for forensic psychotherapy to apply to larger sectors of the community are supported by internationally well-known psychoanalysts such as Kernberg (2014) and Twemlow (2013). Forensic psychotherapy may also contribute to understanding the widespread sexual abuse perpetrated by idealised professionals such as the clergy (priests and nuns), teachers (male and female) or high-profile figures in the entertainment industry, which has been recently exposed but had been hidden from public consciousness for so long. It is not just 'them' of course – therapists can also be abusers.

### A personal perspective

Looking at forensic psychotherapy from my own personal professional experience over a 40-year period, it is clear that the understanding of human behaviour has deepened beyond recognition in the last half century. I want to acknowledge the seminal work of two pioneers in the field of forensic psychotherapy, whom I was fortunate to work with and who influenced my future career.

After completing medical school in Argentina, I studied at the Menninger School of Psychiatry in Topeka, KS, USA. Dr Karl Menninger believed that punishment neither helps the criminal nor protects society.

> Regardless of its futility and expense, punishing criminals gratifies, comforts, and even delights the general public: sadistic attacks in the name of righteousness deal with the public's unconscious guilt about their projective identifications, having conveniently located their aggressive impulses in the criminal, the 'other'. (Menninger, 1967, p. 333)

At the time of the assassination of President Kennedy, Menninger had been devoting his attention to the neglected 'weaker fellowman'. In this instance it was Oswald, the man responsible for President Kennedy's assassination. Menninger stated:

> Thwarted in repeated efforts to have someone pay attention to his puffed up insignificance, this nonentity had concealed himself in a warehouse whence he could overlook thousands of his despised fellow citizens. Far below him they were singing hosannas to their radiant, beloved young leader … The little man in the warehouse was no longer anonymous. (Menninger, 1967, p. 333)

Akhtar's concept of the 'mental pain of the minorities' describes this process aptly as 'In terms of being perceived by the majority, the minority feels both the anguish of invisibility and the torment of hyper-visibility … If one is not wanted but does exist, then what is one to do with one's existence?' (Akhtar, 2014, p. 144)

Menninger's understanding of the single, insignificant man and his position in a society where he was despised and ignored resonates with many current issues that give rise to great concern, even perhaps the terrorist. In this regard, I find it extremely helpful to refer back to the assertion by Gilligan (1996) that a subjective feeling of being humiliated invariably precedes any acts of violence, especially those considered to be 'irrational'. Doctor further elucidates,

> … Even the most apparently insane violence has a meaning in the mind of the person who commits it. There is a need to be aware of this meaning and to learn from it in an attempt to prevent further violence. (Doctor, 2008, p. 2)

From De Zulueta (2006) we have learnt the almost inevitable process that takes place in between mental and physical pain and its development into physical violence. Where De Zulueta makes reference to individual situations, Meloy and Yakeley (2014) apply a similar approach within the context of group and social violence, including acts of genocide and terrorism, which are of topical importance now.

When I left Topeka in 1964 and went to the UK, I worked in one of the most exciting and revolutionary clinical institutions: the Henderson Hospital in London. Dr Maxwell Jones, the second person whom had a major influence on my professional development, had founded this residential unit, or 'therapeutic community' (Jones, 1953), with the aim of treating people with severe personality disorders. I had already met Jones at the Menninger when he came in 1963 to lecture us on his creation of the therapeutic community and we were all deeply impressed by his searching for dignity and social justice for those who, at that point, were called psychopaths and sociopaths.

The enormous challenge of their treatment was met by a sound structure of democracy and the division of labour, in which everyone, patients and staff, shared not only the burden of their treatment but also the administration of the hospital. Admission and discharge procedures reflected part of a philosophy where patients had not only their say, but also could help make decisions regarding the discharge of their peers. Group psychotherapy is a central component of much psychotherapeutic work in a forensic setting and has remained a strong part of my clinical work.

I subsequently obtained a position at the Portman Clinic where I worked until my retirement, 30 years later. I was able to conceptualise my clinical findings about the main characteristics of perversions and was able to focus on the still unreported cases of maternal abuse towards their children. I am very grateful to all those who taught me, especially my patients. The last part of this article will be a discussion of some of that work.

The UK has, from a very early stage, been in the forefront of forensic psychotherapy and, within the UK, the Portman Clinic has been the leader. The history of the Clinic (Rumney, 1981) goes back to 1931, when a small group of men and women psychoanalysts met in London and established an association to promote a better way of dealing with criminals than putting them in prison. It was later called 'The Association for the Scientific Treatment of Delinquency and Crime', a title proposed by an eminent psychoanalyst, Dr Glover, who became its first chairman (Cordess, 1992).

In 1991, while attending a conference of Law and Psychiatry in Belgium, a few colleagues and I discussed how we could foster an understanding of what psychotherapy had to offer to the forensic field. We reached agreement with colleagues from the Netherlands, UK and Switzerland to create our own group, the International Association for Forensic Psychotherapy (IAFP), which adapted the original aims of the English organisation. The IAFP is still going strong and the 24th Annual Conference in 2015 was held at Yale University in the USA, attracting delegates from nine countries. Our next 25th conference will take place in Ghent, Belgium, the very country where the IAFP was born.

Barely a year before the inception of the IAFP, in 1990, the first Course on Forensic Psychotherapy, sponsored by the British Post Graduate Medical Federation, whose director was Professor Michael Peckham at the University of London, in association with the Portman Clinic began to train national and international professionals in the techniques of this special branch of psychotherapy. Our scope was an ambitious one, acknowledging the basic importance of working in a multi-disciplinary way.

I would now like to focus on some of the clinical aspects of forensic psychotherapy that I developed in my work at the Portman Clinic, a National Health Service out-patient clinic (now part of the Tavistock and Portman NHS Foundation Trust), which offers psychoanalytic psychotherapy – both individual and group – to patients presenting with difficulties related to violence, delinquency, criminality or perversion.

## Assessment

In order to assess whether psychotherapy might help an offender we modify some concepts from those used in assessing neurotic patients. Not every offender warrants psychotherapy, not everyone wants it and not everyone benefits. At the Portman Clinic patients are referred from two sources – external and self-referral. External sources include psychiatrists and other professionals working in mental health services, general practitioners, probation officers, courts and other institutions. In some cases public knowledge of a patient's sexual and/or criminal offence is widespread, as a result of that person having appeared in Court, often with associated press reports.

Usually people who refer themselves (both men and women) are those whose 'bizarre' unlawful sexual behaviours are unknown to anyone except themselves and their victims. They come to the Clinic of their own free will. An important characteristic in determining the prognosis and motivation for treatment is whether they have an intense sense of shame and despondency about these activities.

It is important to make a distinction (if possible) between offenders whose criminal activities are ego-dystonic, in other words cause them some degree of mental distress, and those for whom these activities are ego-syntonic. Offenders who have a professional orientation towards their criminal activities may calculate the consequences, such as how many months or years in prison they are prepared to risk. In other words, such offenders may not differ in important psychological traits from careerists generally, and will be less amenable to treatment.

The assessment setting and surroundings are important – especially since the forensic patient has usually had previous experience of the judicial system, having been caught, detected and judged. In his or her dealing with the psychotherapist, the patient is prone to feel judged, charged, persecuted, and subject to prejudice. A new confrontation may well be experienced by the prospective patient as a further condemnation of his or her illegal action. Patients should therefore be treated with dignity and everything reasonable done to give them enough self-respect to face the complexities of their first diagnostic consultation with an unknown consultant.

The patient should be clear from the start the reasons for the assessment interviews, including confidentiality issues, especially if a court report is to be completed. Given the complexity, the assessment process often takes three or four meetings. The 'structuring of time' (Cox, 1992) is a vital frame in forensic psychotherapy and may be different from forensic psychiatry per se. Developing a therapeutic alliance to work together in psychotherapy means a strict adherence to time boundaries. Nevertheless these diagnostic meetings should be conducted at irregular intervals, in order to minimise the intensity of any emerging transference.

During the assessment sessions, there may well be (usually unconscious) attempts to recreate the original injurious, traumatic situation as experienced by the patient. Frequently this will have been experienced as being treated as a 'part-object', and becomes vividly alive in the transference. The establishment of boundaries is crucial to establish a sense of differentiation, in which separating 'them' and 'us' creates a sense of order and justice that can be rightly acknowledged. This is one reason why patients powerfully resent the 'do-gooders' who are seen as trying to proselytise, to infantilise, to make them believe 'we are all the same' – a statement which is felt to be hypocritical, and based on double-standards. The patient who feels guilty does not want his offences to be treated lightly or condoned.

The psychodynamic formulation requires a wide understanding of all the factors concerning that particular person, his psychological growth, his family (going back at least three generations), his subculture, and other circumstances. The psychotherapist needs to investigate the offences in detail, especially the sequence of events leading up to the action as well as the offender's reaction to it. It is important to record how the patient interacts with the clinician and at times it is useful to make a 'trial' interpretation to elicit the patient's capacity to make use of it and his capacity for insight.

Who should be offered individual therapy and who would be best treated in a group? Patients who have never experienced satisfactory relationships in early life, for example those who come from very large families with financial deprivation and emotional overcrowding are likely to do better in individual treatment than in group treatment. Patients who are adopted or fostered react in quite different fashions depending on whether they join a new group in which all members were 'born' simultaneously, or a pre-existing group with a previous history and traditions. In the latter, they may feel 'on trial' and closely observed by the other group members, who are perceived as the 'older', 'legitimate', 'real' children.

Sometimes patients present themselves as 'perfect', 'ideal' patients for group therapy, but it transpires that they are rather good actors, often having been exposed previously to similar experiences in therapeutic prisons or communities. Indeed, they may become good helpers but get little for themselves. This does not mean that they should not be treated in groups, but they warrant special consideration and might be treated more effectively in one-to-one psychotherapy.

Extreme secretiveness is sometimes a contraindication for group therapy. For example, Mr A, who came to the Clinic because of frotteurism, was a shy, awkward, married man with children who had never confessed to anyone about this perversion, and had even refused to give his address. At the first session, when he admitted to his problem, the group's reaction seemed one of anxiety, covered by laughter. Everyone tried to minimise his symptom to such an extent that he felt humiliated, whereupon he became very flushed and left, never to return.

People who have been subjected to an intense, suffocating relationship with one parent may be suitable candidates for group therapy. Groups provide them with a less threatening atmosphere than they can usually find in one-to-one therapy. They can also share their experience with their peers. Often these people are still subjugated to an over-possessive mother, who will not allow them to develop any independence or individuation. Others have managed to leave home only to find themselves extremely isolated. In the group, with the help of fellow patients, they may begin to express openly some rebellious, anti-authority feelings and eventually some self-assertion.

Violent behaviour seems better contained within the framework of group therapy: there is a general tendency to spare those with whom one is identified. The presence of other participants, who may notice hostility before it is expressed openly (often against the therapist), gives the group a capacity to confront violent behaviour and to deal with it openly and honestly. The multiple transferences that exist within the group provide patients with the possibility of more than just one target for their anger, which they find reassuring.

Gaining insight and communicating it are often not that straightforward in working with destructive patients.

### *Case example*

> 'Hector' (notorious for his criminal activities) told the group he was worried about himself:
>
> When I'm about to embark on conning other people I lose my cool. For example, the other day when I went to the bank to pass some forged cheques I got scared. My heart began to pound, I got all sweaty in my hands, I avoided eye to eye contact with the cashier. In other words, I was giving myself away.

Another member asked, 'Do you think this consciousness has anything to do with this group?' Everybody showed much interest in this statement, to which he replied, 'Yes. It has all happened since I came here and I am very scared'. This was an important change, which had to do with his criminal activity changing from ego-syntonic to ego-dystonic. In other words, his capacity to corrupt his ego integrity was no longer so easily available, due to the formation of a new ego, which had been internalised from the group, with an accompanying capacity for reflection. The group was split in two: some accepted this as a healthy development, but others were not as generous with their response because of envy. One member, said,

> I am extremely worried about you and the effect this group has on you if this means that you are becoming more ineffectual as a thief. Perhaps you ought to do something about that – I don't know whether you ought to leave the group or what, but be sure that the group is not affecting your skills as a thief.

Others in the group reacted to this statement angrily, calling it cynical. They pointed out that after all Hector had come to therapy in order to deal with his criminal actions. His challenger was merciless with his manic reaction, saying while laughing:

> He's not coming here to deal with his thieving problems, he's coming here because, as the doctor has remarked on many occasions, of his sense of emptiness, his deadness and his looking for excitement. So, first he'll have to know about this boredom. In the meantime he has to be careful not to get caught.

## The treatment setting

Because of their fears of intimacy in the one-to-one situation patients often form a strong transference to the Clinic as an institution. One crucial point about the discipline of forensic psychotherapy is that it is usually a team effort involving a wide range of people. Successful treatment rests not only with the specialist psychoanalytical psychotherapist, who will be from one of a number of core professions such as psychiatry, psychology, nursing, social work or the creative arts, but also with a team of helpers, including managers, administrators and clerical staff who get involved with the patient at all levels and in different settings.

When it comes to treatment, forensic patients are very much in need of four structures; fellow patients, therapist, institution and family (if they have one). An important function provided by the institution is that of containment in the psychological as well as the literal sense. The institution reinforces a sense of boundaries and so acts as a container for all tensions involved and allows the emergence of trust and a collective awareness of, and sensitivity to, the recrudescence of violence, thus reducing its likelihood. The staff should themselves feel safe and securely contained in caring and unobtrusive surroundings, to reduce the inherent anxiety produced by working with forensic patients. The patients can act out sadistic and intrusive attacks on therapists and on their treatment in many different ways, including on their capacity to think; this leaves therapists confused and unable to offer adequate interpretations. At times of crisis, when for many reasons staff members are unable to fulfil their tasks properly, a breakdown of the system is likely – with serious consequences for all, including the patients. Adlam et al. (2012), in their book *The Therapeutic Milieu Under Fire*, described the different problems facing the multi-professional staff in different settings, and the ways of containing anxiety. This includes music therapy, which has been shown to be effective in prisons and other safety places for offenders (Compton et al., 2012).

**Transference and counter-transference**

Forensic psychotherapy patients have experienced – as infants – a sense of having been messed about in crucial circumstances in which both their psychological and biological survival were at stake. In other words they were actually – in reality, not only in fantasy, – at the mercy of others. These traumatic, continuous and inconsistent attitudes towards them have effectively interfered with the process of individuation and separation. There is a basic lack of trust towards the significant carer, which accompanies them all through their lives and will colour their experience of therapy.

Elaborate and sophisticated unconscious mechanisms have been built-up that operate as a 'self-survival kit': this is 'turned on' automatically in situations of extreme vulnerability when they experience being psychically naked or 'stripped'. For example over-sexualisation can be a means of dealing with an enormous sense of inadequacy and of inner insecurity. It is obvious that all these different survival mechanisms and ways of functioning will appear intermittently when their defences are down. Old feelings of alarm re-emerge and put the person concerned on the alert. The one-way system has become a two-way system that is in constant dynamic activity.

Defence mechanisms go in waves and when a situation of closeness is about to be achieved the person may withdraw in horror. Such people loathe any new scenario, which might involve or develop into trust. The neutral therapist is experienced as a tyrannical and despotic parental figure, who is only there to satisfy his/her own whims. The task for the therapist is to gradually help the person work through such painful feelings. 'The forensic psychotherapist spends much of his time and energy waiting and witnessing, while his patients try to unravel that vitally important nodal point of experience 'between the acting of a dreadful thing/And the first motion' (Cox, 1992).

The psychotherapist must listen to the patient carefully, without interrupting, however difficult or painful the material may be. This is frequently the case with incestuous relationships. It is important to be aware of how our own feelings may be the origin, for example, of the under-recording of female perversions such as female paedophilia and maternal incest. Patients may be ready to talk about these urges but diagnosticians generally are not ready to listen to them. The requirement of personal therapy for future therapists is of basic importance, in order to be able to discern what belongs to our internal world and what to the patient's. Much of these patients' material can disturb us profoundly because at times it feels like dealing with 'dynamite' (Welldon, 2011). Sometimes, if unprepared, the therapist may become irate, as if he or she is being 'taken for a ride', or the patient is trying to be in total control of the situation. In other instances, patients succeed in making their therapists become their true partners in their specific perversions.

### *Case example*

A patient came for a diagnostic interview because of his compulsive masochistic needs. These involved hiring prostitutes to actively ill-treat him in a way that sexually excited him. In the course of the interview, the therapist found to her horror that she had become actively engaged in a dialogue in which she began to scream at the top of her voice. She realised that every time she tried to say something to the patient he asked her to repeat it 'just a bit louder, because I'm hard of hearing'. One of the reasons the therapist became aware of her own response was that at the time the patient was relating an incident in which he had secured the services of a nurse to function as a sadistic prostitute. The nurse symbolised the therapeutic situation, which had been corrupted.

Alternatively, the therapist may feel flattered by the fact that whatever positive change may have been achieved, the patient ascribes it to the practitioner's own professional work. However, the flattery won't last for long; it will soon be replaced by complaints and dissatisfaction about relapses or re-offending now assumed to be due to the practitioner's inefficiency and lack of 'skills', just as before the 'cure' of the problem had to do with his/her excellence. In other words, there is a constant switch between idealisation and denigration. This happens because psycho-pathological predicaments and offending behaviour are often the result of a deep, chronic, hidden depression. This may become manifest in a manic and at times bizarrely funny acting out. Although patients try at all costs to avoid their real feelings, there is so much pain underneath that they may barely manage to confront it. The most severe, although not apparently obvious, is that the forensic patient is unable to think before the action occurs because he is not mentally equipped to make the necessary links (Bion, 1959). The therapist can become easily caught in the countertransference process, assuming an omnipotent role in the patient's actions regardless of whether they are law abiding or not.

A relapse in delinquent and criminal behaviour is frequently found during breaks in psychotherapy. This is associated with feelings of having been abandoned by their therapists at times of need. To quote Gallwey (1991):

> The uncovering of areas of deprivation and unfulfilled dependency can produce enormous pressure on both therapist and patient, with a speedy move into delinquent acting out, or even violence, when the patient feels let down or abandoned within

the therapy. The least hazardous tactic is to contain the individual in a way which minimises the reinforcement of delinquent strategies.

## The link between criminal actions and sexual deviations

Often, forensic patients are deviant both sexually and socially. For example, some sexual deviations present themselves as criminal activities by definition, although some patients who indulge in these actions may never have been caught. This is a secret or secretive population who apparently lead normal lives, sometimes in both work and domestic situations. However, the links between criminal actions such as 'breaking and entering' and sexual deviations are not always obvious, at least not until the unconscious motivation is revealed. This connection has been noticed by many psychoanalytical authors, such as Zilboorg (1955), Glover (1944), and notably in young persons by Limentani (1984).

### *Case example*

A young man was referred several years ago to the Portman Clinic by his employers, a City bank. It was, in itself, a revelation that a City bank could be so perceptive of the possibility of unconscious motivations to make this referral, which speaks to the sense of bewilderment the man had caused with his puzzling offence. He was the bank's 'bike man', responsible for carrying money from and to different places. In the course of his work, he had been detected stealing spanners from other bikes' boxes. Alarm grew to great dimensions when police found evidence of his having previously stolen 3000 spanners. At the interview with me he tried unsuccessfully to make sense of his unlawful actions by explaining that he was a handyman and that the price of tools was subject to inflation. Obviously, such a clumsy and inadequate explanation pointed to other motivations. In describing his actions, he talked with a great deal of embarrassment mixed with excitement. In his own words he said:

> I'm on my bike. Suddenly I see another bike being parked and I feel taken over by an extreme curiosity to look at its box. I know this is wrong but cannot help myself. I start sweating. I feel my heart pumping and I just have to do it. I have to take the tools. Then I feel at peace, a great sense of relief surrounds me. I feel great. On my way home I start feeling confused, ashamed and guilty. I don't know any longer what to do with yet another spanner and I take it to the garage where I keep them all.

This patient's statement is similar to that of a person suffering from sexual perversion, showing the same quality of urgency, the identical cycle which involves growing sexual anxiety, the fight against it, eventually giving in and succumbing to the action, the sexual relief, and the subsequent sense of shame and guilt.

This was a young, well-groomed man who was still living with his mother, a domineering narcissistic woman who had never allowed him to lead his own life. When the police came to get him, her first reaction was: 'What shall I do if you take him away. I can't be on my own'. Apart from his mother he had never had any relationship of any sort and lived in complete isolation. Our psychiatric court report briefly indicated that this man's criminal offences were the expression of his tremendous sense of social and sexual inadequacy which, in turn, were the product of a deprived and depraved early childhood. His father had been absent and his mother had a severe narcissistic borderline personality. The magistrate not only found the report but also the recommendation useful. The patient was recommended to seek treatment in group psychotherapy, which if accepted was to be immediately implemented. The work of psychotherapy consisted of his growing awareness of the unconscious links between the sexual symbolisms and the enactment of his irresistible impulses. This unraveling made it possible for the patient to free himself from these urges.

## The overlapping of sexual predicaments and hidden violence

A young man of 23 first came to treatment because of fears of being homosexual. After a year of individual psychotherapy he left treatment having seemingly overcome that particular problem. A few years later, however, he was back, this time, because he had experienced sudden, and unexpectedly, violent fantasies against all women, but particularly his mother, and later on his girl friend. He had achieved an intimate situation with his girlfriend but had felt the urge to hurt her. In an obvious attempt to do so, he had had a one-night stand with another girl. He started group therapy and in one session described a recent dream in which he had his fist inside a woman's vagina and was punching it vigorously. When he began to enjoy this process he became aware that he was disintegrating; first the hand began to dissolve and later the whole body was annihilated. This dream represented his fears of being destroyed by a woman if he became close to her. His fear of homosexuality had been a protection – replaced later by a deeper fear, expressed through violent fantasies – against women who he felt had previously damaged him, indeed almost emasculated him.

## The different aims of male and female perversions

As a clinician I have observed that the main difference between a male and female perverse action lies in the aim. Whereas in men the act is aimed at an outside part-object, in women it is usually against themselves, either against their bodies or against objects which they see as their own creations, that is, their babies. In both cases, bodies and babies are treated as part-objects (Welldon, 1988).

### *Case example*

A woman patient was referred because of exhibitionism. She told me that her compulsion to 'flash' occurred when she became attached to a person whom she invested with idealised 'maternal' qualities. She wanted to get closer, to be noticed and to be taken care of by that particular person but she also wanted a shocked response from her 'victims'. She carefully planned the 'appropriate' clothing to wear when she was to meet that person, usually an overcoat covering only a little vest in order to respond readily to her urges. She knew this was wrong and that she would be rejected but she could not stop herself.

She described a most deprived early history of being sexually abused by her mother and her siblings. It is interesting to note that, even when her exhibitionism could superficially appear to be the equivalent of her male counterpart's, this is not so. It is well-documented that male exhibitionists often have the compulsion 'to flash' only to women – and women who are unknown to them – while my patient had suffered from this compulsion only with other women with whom she felt a close attachment. This is yet another remarkable difference between the genders.

### *Case example*

This example is of a patient I treated many years ago and to whom I owe much of my own clarity and expertise in this field. She was a practising prostitute who was referred for a psychiatric assessment because of violent behaviour directed towards her second child. She had been a victim herself of paternal sexual abuse. Her first pregnancy came as a surprise to her. Still, she felt the need to go ahead with it, because in this way she was taking out insurance against a dread of being alone in that the child could become utterly dependent on her and totally under her control. When this first child arrived, she was overcome by feelings of repulsion and revulsion against her baby. She felt ready to kick it, and after reflection she decided that in order to overcome these horrid feelings she would fix in her mind the idea of the baby being part of herself. Some days she would choose her right arm as being the baby, and at other times it would be one of her legs. In this way she felt able to master her impulses to beat up her first child. Later with her second baby she asserted, 'There is no more room in my body for a second one. All has been used up by the first one'.

## Conclusion

In this article I have described the history of forensic psychotherapy and my own involvement in its development. Now in its second century, forensic psychotherapy has a long and rich history that should be celebrated. It is a serious academic and clinical discipline that provides us with a unified theory of psychopathology, a clear model of assessment, and treatment with a coherent philosophy of compassion (hope with expertise). It has grown and flourished from a minority interest to a full fledged profession. However, it has still greater potential for growth through more publications, through longitudinal research and through the creation of formal institutional structures such as training programmes and dedicated salaried posts for forensic psychotherapy in both health and criminal justice settings.

## Disclosure statement

No potential conflict of interest was reported by the author.

## References


Adlam, J., Aiyegbusi, A., Kleinot, P., Motz, A., & Scanlon, C. (2012). *The therapeutic milieu under fire: Security and insecurity in forensic mental health.* London: Jessica Kingsley Publishers.

Aiyegbusi, A., & Kelly, G. (Eds.). (2012). *Professional and therapeutic boundaries in forensic mental health practice.* London: Jessica Kingsley Publishers.

Akhtar, S. (2014). The mental pain of minorities. *British Journal of Psychotherapy, 30,* 136–153.

Altshul, V. A. (2013). Commentary: Forensic psychotherapy. *Journal of American Academy of Psychiatry Law, 41,* 46–48.

Bion, W. R. (1959). Attacks on linking. *International Journal of Psychoanalysis, 40,* 308–315.

Bluglass, R. (1990). The scope of forensic psychiatry. *Journal of Forensic Psychiatry, 1,* 7.

Cordess, C. (1992). Pioneers in forensic psychiatry. *Journal of Forensic Psychiatry, 3,* 509–530.

Cox, M. (1992). Forensic Psychotherapy: an emergent discipline. In *Proceedings of the 17th International Congress of the International Academy of Law and Mental Health,* Leuven, Belgium (p. 338).

Curen, R., & Sinason, V. (2010). Learning-disabled adults and children. In C. Itzin, A. Taket, & S. Barter-Godfrey (Eds.), *Domestic and sexual violence and abuse: Tackling the health and mental health effects* (pp. 132–138). Abingdon: Routledge.

De Zulueta, F. (2006). *From pain to violence: The Traumatic Roots of Destructiveness.* (2nd ed.). Chichester: Whurr Publishers.

Doctor, R. (Ed.). (2008). *Murder: A psychotherapeutic investigation.* London: Karnac Books.

Freud, S. (1915). Some character-types met with in psycho-analytic work. *Standard Edition, 14,* 311–333.

Gallwey, P. (1991). Social maladjustment. In J. Holmes (Ed.), *Textbook of psychotherapy in psychiatric practice.* London: Churchills Livingstone.

Gilligan, J. (1996). *Violence: Reflections on our deadliest epidemic.* New York, NY: Grosset/Putnam Books.

Glover, E. (1944). "*The diagnosis and treatment of delinquency*" *Mental Abnormality and Crime* (pp. 269–299). London: Macmillan & Co.

Glover, E. (1960). *The roots of crime.* London: Imago.

Harding, T. (1992). *Research and evaluation in forensic psychotherapy.* Presented at 1st International Conference of the International Association of Forensic Psychotherapy, London.

Hopper, E. (1991). Encapsulation as a defence against the fear of annihilation. *International Journal of Psychoanalysis, 72,* 607–624.

Jones, M. (1953). *The therapeutic community: A new treatment method in psychiatry*. New York, NY: Basic Books.
Kernberg, O. (2014). Innovation in psychoanalytic education. *New Associations, 16*, 10–11.
Limentani, A. (1984). Toward a unified conception of the origins of sexual and social deviancy in young persons. *International Journal of Psychoanalytic Psychotherapy, 10*, 383–401.
Meloy, J. R. & Yakeley, J. (2014). The violent true believer as a 'Lone Wolf' - Psychoanalytic Perspectives on Terrorism, *Behavioural Sciences & the Law, 32*, 347–365.
Menninger, K. (1967). The injustice of justice: Who is to blame? *Bulletin of the Menninger Clinic, 31*, 325–333.
Pfäfflin, F. (1992). What is in a symptom? A conservative approach in the therapy of sex offenders. *Journal of Offender Rehabilitation, 18*, 5–17.
Reed report. (1992). Department of Health/Home Office Report of the Academic Advisory Group.
Ronson, J. (2015). *So you've been publically shamed*. London: Picador.
Rumney, D. (1981). Unpublished monograph.
Sinason, V. (2010). *Mental handicap and the human condition: An analytic approach to intellectual disability. Second updated edition*. London: Free Association Books.
Tuovinen (1973). *Crime as an attempt at intrapsychic adaptation*. Oulu, Finland: University of Oulu.
Twemlow, S., Sacco, F., & Williams, P. (1996). A clinical and interactionist perspective on the bully-victim-bystander relationship. *Bulletin of the Menninger Clinic, 60*, 296–313.
Twemlow, S. (2013). Broadening the vision: A case for community-based psychoanalysis in the context of usual practice. *Journal of the American Psychoanalytic Association, 61*, 662–690.
Welldon, E. V. (1984). The application of group analytic psychotherapy to those with sexual perversions. In Lear T. E. (Ed.) *Spheres of group analysis* (pp. 96–108). Naas, Co. Kildare: Leicester Leader Ltd.
Welldon, E. (1988). *Mother, Madonna, Whore: The idealisation and denigration of motherhood*. London: Free Association Books. [American Edition, Guilford Press, 1992. Current edition UK, Karnac, 2004].
Welldon, E. V. (2011). *Playing with dynamite: A personal approach to the psychoanalytic understanding of perversion, violence and criminality*. London: Karnac.
Williams, T. (1991). *Forensic psychotherapy: Symbiosis or impossibility*. Presented at 17th International Congress of the International Academy of Law and Mental Health, Leuven, Belgium.
Winnicott, D. W. (1956). The Antisocial Tendency. In *Collected Papers: Through Pediatrics to Psychoanalysis (1975)* (pp. 306–315). London: Hogarth Press.
Yakeley, J., & Adshead, G. (2013). Locks, keys, and security of mind: Psychodynamic approaches to forensic psychiatry. *The Journal of the American Academy of Psychiatry and the Law, 41*, 38–45.
Zilboorg, G. (1955). *The psychology of the criminal act and punishment*. London: Hogarth Press & Institute of Psychoanalysis.

# Female violence and toxic couples

Anna Motz

*Oxford Clinic, Littlemore Mental Health Centre, Littlemore,Oxford, UK*

The author describes the development and expression of violence by women against their own children and against their partners, within a perverse relationship, or 'toxic coupling'. Female aggression against intimate partners can be a feature of these relationships, playing a significant role in the perpetuation of destructive interactions. The fact of female violence in such partnerships is often minimised or denied altogether and the male is identified as the perpetrator while the female is configured simply as the victim: the author describes how such a view of women reflects a failure to acknowledge the reality of female agency and perversion. This, in turn, prevents a full understanding of the complex dynamics of violent relationships and effective psychotherapeutic interventions with them, leaving children exposed to such situations at serious risk. This concept rests on the notion that it is not the individual partners that are 'toxic' but the relationship itself, with its entrenched destructive dynamics. The 'toxic couple' is created by the interaction of two disturbed individual attachment systems in each, revealing the violent impulses and psychic disturbance of the female as well as the male partner. In this paper, the author describes how women, as well as their male partners, can be both perpetrators and victims of extreme cruelty. As with female violence generally, because females are assumed not to be violent, there is a danger that some aspects of toxic partnerships are so taboo as to be unthinkable.

## Introduction: female violence and toxic couples

The field of forensic psychotherapy has offered tremendous insight into how the dual role of perpetrator and victim can coexist in the same person, and demonstrated the unconscious motivations that underlie serious acts of violence. These include the wish to be caught and punished out of a sense of unconscious guilt as described by Freud in 1916:

> Paradoxical as it may sound, I must maintain that the sense of guilt was present before the misdeed, that it did not arise from it, but conversely – the misdeed arose from the sense of guilt. These people might justly be described as criminals from a sense of guilt. The pre-existence of the guilty feeling had of course been

> demonstrated by a whole set of other manifestations and effects. (Freud, 1916, p. 332)

The desire for containment and punishment can lead offenders to commit their crimes clumsily, as if seeking to be caught, and to express a profound sense of relief when this occurs, and they are subsequently punished. The inner world of the forensic patient has been described in rich detail (e.g. Glasser, 1979; Morgan, 2007), in terms of violent and perverse enactments, shaping psychotherapeutic work with men in settings as diverse as prisons, probation settings and outpatient clinics. The Portman Clinic in London is often credited as the birthplace of this thinking, with an important educational and training function. According to its model of forensic psychotherapy, an analysis of the offence can uncover the psychic conflicts of the individual, analogous to the symptom in a neurotic condition; unlike traditional psychoanalysis it gives the role of society in relation to the inner world of the offender a central place. (Welldon, 1996)

This understanding has also been extended to address the roots and expressions of violence and perversion in women, and to challenge the assumption that this occurs in only the rarest of cases. In her seminal work on female perversion, Welldon (1988) introduced the notion of maternal perversion and described the narcissistic use of children to extend a woman's own maltreatment of her body, and to repeat an intergenerational pattern of abuse and cruelty. She challenged the assumption that a phallus was an essential prerequisite of perversion and shocked clinicians with her startling and unsettling discoveries about the potential for mothers to use their own bodies and those of their children in the service of perverse activity. She offers an extensive description of the characteristics of female perversion in her early and later work (Welldon, 1988, 2011).

For women, as for men, the meaning of the offence is not necessarily accessible to the conscious mind, but becomes clearer throughout the course of analytic psychotherapy, manifested through the relationship with the therapist. For this to take place successfully, the therapist must retain neutrality, openness and an acute awareness of the danger of re-enactments.

## Female violence and intimate relationships

In this paper, I explore female violence in the context of destructive, perverse and violent partnerships that I refer to as toxic couples. This violence can be understood as a reflection of unconscious forces, often in direct contradiction to what is consciously wanted. Although such violence can be dramatically expressed against her partner, her children or the woman herself, it is often hidden from view, enacted in secret in the private domain of the home, and in unseen places on the bodies or on victims who can not or will not speak about it. Its hidden, clandestine nature is mirrored in the societal response, which is often to deny the fact of such violence altogether, whether in relation to maternal abuse or female aggression within intimate relationships.

I will discuss the role of female violence within abusive relationships, focussing on those couples whose attraction is based on malignant forces, often unconscious, but always compelling. These perverse couplings can be highly addictive and the bond between the pair appears to be based on a shared need to engage in abusive practices (Welldon, 2002). At times the perverse activity of the couple extends to their own children, or those of others, viewed largely as objects to be used for their own gratification. I will discuss clinical situations in which women were violent within what I have called 'toxic couples' and describe in some detail how this impacts on the therapy

Although we often think of domestic violence as perpetrated by one person, usually a male perpetrator, against a victim (often female), I suggest that within a toxic relationship it is the interaction of the two individuals that creates this destructive force, even when one partner is the principal enactor of the violence. Within some such relationships the woman herself is the primary aggressor, using her partner as an object onto which to project her own feelings of disgust, humiliation and unworthiness. He in turn becomes the 'poison container', filled with shame and a sense of degradation (deMause, 1990). Sometimes women unconsciously locate their own aggressive impulses into their partners, and this frees them temporarily from awareness of their own violent wishes towards others. It is even possible to view the attraction of some women to violent partners, who abuse them, as a form of self-harm, in that their partners enact their own savage impulses towards themselves.

Aggression and intimacy can be inextricably interwoven in these relationships, to the extent that the currency of communication is itself violent: a kiss with a fist. I explore this dangerous dance, revealing the conscious and unconscious dynamics of violence between partners, and its alarming complexity (Motz, 2014).

All kinds of couples can become enmeshed in destructive dynamics, with the potential for serious harm against one another and/or any children within the family. The role of both partners in the dangerous and compelling patterns of interacting that underpin violent relationships requires analysis, and their respective contributions disentangled.

The nature of the bond between women who have been sexually abused and their abuser can be seen as a malignant attachment – this is clearly the case in incestuous relationships, where a child or adolescent has been forced or seduced into a sexual relationship with a parent or sibling. When these abusive relationships are re-created in later life, women as well as men can inflict serious levels of harm on one another, and on children within their household. The consequences of incest are profound for both male and female children, but the stigma of female sex offending can make it difficult for boys to disclose their abuse, especially if members of their own families are perpetrators. This is a gross example of a toxic coupling that has destructive effects, both immediately in the long term As in other cases of child abuse and trauma, a woman who has been abused early in life may go on to perpetrate a similar violation against another, perhaps only many years later. In so doing she acts in identification with the aggressor (A. Freud, 1936) and attempts to rid herself of shameful and unwanted feelings by treating another person as she herself has been treated. I will turn now to a clinical illustration of this process, where the chosen objects of abuse and humiliation are a male partner, and a female child.

### *Clinical vignette: between a volcano and a void*

When I met her, Paula was 42 years old, referred for psychotherapy because of her long history of violence against others, including her partner, her children and various mental health professionals whom she had stalked and threatened. She had a diagnosis of borderline personality disorder, and been hospitalised on numerous occasions. These admissions had resulted only in further deterioration in her mental health and were characterised by her assaults on staff and frequent 'restraints' which she appeared both to invite and resist. She had been rejected for outpatient treatment by mainstream mental health services because of her violence, and was subsequently referred to the forensic psychotherapy and psychology service.[1]

At assessment Paula was rather withdrawn and flat, presenting as emotionally 'shut down' but with sudden flashes of liveliness, that took me by surprise. She conveyed a powerful sense of discomfort and suppressed violence, so I felt I needed to tread gently. Early on she told me about her struggle with feeling she was 'female' as she tended to regard herself as masculine. She felt she did not possess femininity as she associated this with vulnerability, softness and helplessness. She suddenly commented that she felt that I was 'comfortable' with my femininity and told me she would never be able to wear a skirt or high-heeled shoes, as I was. At this moment I felt suddenly exposed and judged in a harsh fashion, and that there was an implicit accusation in her comment. Her statement highlighted our differences and also that we were two women, together in an intimate therapeutic encounter. I felt that her sudden and sharp comment was unconsciously designed to throw me off balance, and to raise a question about my version of 'femininity'. This gave me an important insight into her distrust of me, and how quickly her mood and perceptions changed. Despite her suspicions, she felt able to tell me about her early life, and her past and present difficulties. Paula felt she was out of control, and was driving her family away with her volatile moods and angry outbursts.

At the end of the three-session assessment, we agreed to work together over a period of eighteen months in weekly psychotherapy. Her violence was not a threat to the general public, but, as is typical of female violence, was targeted towards herself in savage acts of self-harm, her partner, her children, and towards those in a 'caring' position in relation to her, like the psychiatrists she had threatened and the nurses on the wards.

The oldest of four girls, Paula had been subjected to physical harm by her own mother for much of her life and frequently left alone or with unsuitable carers from an early age, to care for her younger siblings. Additionally, and significantly, an older male relative, in whose care she had often been left as a small girl, sometimes with her siblings and sometimes entirely alone, had sexually abused her. This sexual abuse had continued for several years, beginning when she was six years old and continuing until she was eleven, by which time her abuser was engaging her in penetrative intercourse. Paula's attempts to tell her parents were met with disbelief and indifference. She had a troubled adolescence, displaying aggression to others at school, alongside sexual promiscuity, substance misuse and cruelty to animals. At 16, she formed an attachment to young man several years older, and later married him. He was devoted to her but suffered from depression and intermittent substance misuse, himself the only child of a mother who was an addict, and who had been physically violent to him during his childhood. Paula became pregnant with their daughter when she was 18. Her partner promised to support her to care for the baby. Paula hated the feelings of discomfort, nausea and heaviness that she experienced during pregnancy, and the sense of being invaded by an alien creature; it was only her strong belief that abortion was wrong that prevented her from terminating the pregnancy. After childbirth, she had found the care of her baby girl intolerable and became withdrawn and angry, feeling that she had been robbed of her freedom and that her body had been destroyed by both the pregnancy and the labour, which left her feeling 'torn apart and broken'. The pregnancy had been unplanned.

She had later had a second baby, a son, to whom she felt far closer, enjoying a loving bond that she had not been able to establish with her daughter. Paula described her guilt feelings about her violence towards her partner, and her physical abuse and neglect of her children, particularly her daughter. Despite her palpable sense of shame, she was articulate and insightful as she recalled her disgust with her daughter's constant need for feeding and described a powerful sense of persecution related to what she perceived to be her insatiable needs. She described a sense of guilt about this estrangement and recognised that she treated her daughter much as she herself had been treated, with a degree of cruelty and a wish to be rid of her. Her partner, like Paula's own father, was the more affectionate and stable parent, which she both envied and valued. Acknowledging this painful mix of feelings was difficult for her.

Although Paula had enjoyed some time with her son, she noted that her volatile mood swings had worsened with the birth of each child and she found herself alternating between self-harming and violent assaults on others, sparing him. Her partner, who was effectively the main carer for both their children, subsequently became the target of her rage. He, in turn, withdrew into greater substance and alcohol misuse, generally at night time when the children were asleep, and when she would discover this, she would physically assault him. As the relationship grew more volatile he sought solace in friendships with other women, which he claimed were not sexual but offered comfort in his loneliness and shame. These associations, in turn, fuelled Paula's sense of rage, jealousy and underlying feelings of abandonment. Her violence towards him became more frequent and also more severe, and he would sometimes retaliate through physical aggression. Their relationship became a fraught and violent, as their fights escalated, and, on occasion, it seemed to Paula that her partner was taunting her with evidence of his intimacy with other women, as though goading her into a jealous frenzy. Her own terror of abandonment and wish to control her partner, led her into becoming an 'intimate partner terrorist' (Johnson, 2008) who wanted to exert her will on every aspect of her partner's life. Unsurprisingly the needs of their young children were neglected within this toxic coupling.

Paula spent much of the early part of the work describing how she would take out her anger on her daughter, alternating between physical abuse of her, and neglect, demonstrating what I have termed an oscillation between 'the volcano and the void'. Her daughter became clingy, distrustful and markedly unhappy, in contrast to her son, who remained rather more settled, apparently confident in his mother's love, but fearful of the violent rows he witnessed between his parents. Paula found her daughter's clinginess and anxious outbursts when she left her persecutory, seeing them as evidence that she was 'an unfit mother', and avoided time with her. She told me that at one level she had been, aware at of the harm she was inflicting on her, but, at another, had turned 'a blind eye' to the cruelty to which she subjected her. This seemed to be her way of defending herself from acknowledging her violence towards her daughter, with whom she powerfully, and destructively, identified. Over the course of therapy she also described vivid memories of emotional and physical violence between her parents and her mother's physical assaults on her.

## Countertransference issues

It was clear that there was a risk of becoming another 'toxic couple' with Paula, and having the therapy become a hostage to her assaults on the work. She and I needed to find a way of collaborating and enabling the therapeutic space to be one in which thoughtful exploration could take place, rather than an intense, fraught environment that relied on actions rather than emotional engagement. She often arrived at sessions in a highly guarded fashion, and sometimes argued with reception staff on the way in, as though discharging difficult feelings before meeting with me. This put me in the position akin to a child, watching parents fight, and feeling helpless, collusive and slightly frightened. She walked robotically to the room and held herself stiffly, showing me she was 'on guard'. During the course of the treatment, I found myself warding off indirect threats, in the form of attacks on the efficacy of the work or through elaborated fantasies of what she would like to inflict on other professionals, and on people who let her down. I was in her good books, but I was aware how quickly, and dramatically, this could switch. In her rigid paranoid-schizoid functioning, it was impossible for her to hold the awareness of mixed feelings in mind, or to forgive me my imperfections. In this sense I did feel a hostage, frightened to miss a session or show any kind of weakness, but was able to interpret this to her, as it showed us clearly how intolerant she was of any vulnerability of her own.

At other times I was left in anxious suspense, told about the violent feelings that Paula had towards neighbours, her husband and herself, and her wishes to act on them. As her children had left home, I was not distracted by child protection worries, though her treatment of them in the past had been of serious concern, as she herself acknowledged. She was adamant that she did not want to engage in couple therapy with her husband and that she only wanted this individual therapy with me.

At times I felt quite battered by her, and scared to speak, but when I suggested to her that she was communicating her wish to silence me, alongside her hope that I would be able to bear her anger and threats, she softened and became accessible to exploring her own fears of vulnerability, shame and abandonment. I felt that I needed to summon up all my strength and courage to confront the power of her intimidation and aggressive and destructive feelings conveyed through a real threat of violence in the room. It seemed essential that I could bear and articulate this, but it was, at times, difficult for me to keep this thought alive. The unconscious wish for me to stay strong and thoughtful was in sharp contrast to her conscious challenges to me, and the threatening manner of her direct, personal questions to me. At times, I felt in identification with her frightened husband, and the children who had both relied on and feared her.

At other times, I found myself anxious before her sessions, almost hoping she might miss them, which she never did, and this alerted me to the sense in which I could become as neglectful and abandoning as her own mother. The part of me that wished her away, for my own peace of mind, was in clear identification with her rejecting parent, and also informed my understanding of her sense of being unwanted, unloved and unworthy. It would not have been difficult to repeat the pattern of other services and reject her out of fear, and an unconscious wish to retaliate against her. When she did appear, I would experience mixed feelings, both apprehensive and relieved, pleased she was able to bring herself to the session and ashamed of my own fear.

During the sessions, Paula would often invite frank appraisals about her physical appearance and describe her discomfort in relation to it, only to become visibly unsettled after asking these questions, and expressing her own self-contempt. I thought that this also put me in the place of someone who looked at her, in an objectifying and potentially desiring manner, as if considering her for sexual use. This seemed to relate to her unconscious need to re-enact a relationship with her own abuser, perhaps in order to 'master the trauma' in the here and now. She was able to think about how she had herself identified with her abuser, treating her body with contempt and retaining a sense of suspicion about herself. We were able to consider how she had internalised him, constantly surveying her own body and then attacking it, through brutal acts of self-harm. I felt that I was unconsciously invited to both participate in and become witness to her perverse self-treatment.

Paula would describe in some detail her attacks on her husband, who seemed to tolerate these, in what seemed a form of masochistic surrender. When she eventually made a clear link between her own parents' violent interactions and how she treated her husband, she seemed to become less wedded to her own aggression, and more in touch with her wish to engage in loving interactions with him. Over the course of the therapy, she gradually reduced her violent assaults on him and she self-harmed less frequently and with less destructive methods. By the time that the therapy ended, she felt less frightening, and less frightened, but still retreated into her world of violent fantasies at times of stress. Interestingly, she controlled the timing of the ending, and chose to leave just short of the 18 months we had originally agreed. Perhaps because her growing sense of vulnerability was too uncomfortable for her. I noted my sense of sadness that this complex and difficult work was ending, in contrast to the apprehension with which I had begun the work.

The development of perversions, including the sadistic use of violence and threats, can be a means of securing a false sense of confidence in one's capacity to manage the threats posed by intimate relationships. The need to control the other is a central feature of perversion and offers the promise that the object will not pose a threat to psychic integrity of the individual, through abandonment or engulfment (Glasser, 1979.) Giving pain felt far safer than facing the risk of receiving it, and returning to a place of humiliation and fear. In the work with Paula, it was essential that I was not pulled into a sado-masochistic relationship but remained able to think with her about the feelings that underlay her violence.

Viewing domestic violence as simply an expression of the male wish for power and control is both reductive and inaccurate. Some feminist analyses risk this when it is accepted unquestioningly, as Dutton and Nicholls (2005) argue in their review of the literature: 'A case is made for a paradigm having developed among family violence activists and researchers that precludes the notion of female violence, trivializes injuries to males and maintains a monolithic view of a complex social problem.' (2005, p. 680). In the following clinical vignette, I describe the particular situation of a woman who hurts her child within the context of a violent relationship.

### *Clinical vignette: Maja*

In some cases of domestic violence, the mother turns her anger against her own children, not simply because of own identification with the battered child, and an expression of her unhappiness, but as a form of revenge, comfort or to draw attention to the crisis of her relationship, by creating a situation in which other agencies become involved. She may be unaware of these unconscious motivations for her actions.

In one such case, a young mother, Maja, came to me for therapy as a result of social services' involvement with her seven-month old baby son. He had suffered a fractured arm, whose causes were determined to be non-accidental. Maja had taken him to hospital and was thought to be a devoted and gentle carer, while her husband, who had a violent history and a criminal record for charges of assault, theft and driving while disqualified, was at first suspected of causing the injuries. Social services responded by placing him on the 'At Risk Register' and recommending to the parents that the father seek anger management and the mother help for depression. Both parents were recent immigrants to the UK and the father had been given legal status when he had arrived as an unaccompanied minor, having then met the mother through friends from the local community of people from their community. Although the mother had a sister here, with whom she had been when she had met her partner, she had little other social or family support in the UK and was isolated, appearing vulnerable and depressed.

Although it was initially difficult to engage her in the therapeutic work, as she seemed so flat and distrustful, she gradually become more alive in the therapy, sustaining eye contact and talking to me about the difficulties of her early life, and her sense of displacement in the UK. She described the violence and control that her husband inflicted on her, and how she wished she could take her son and return to her family home. However, after six sessions she also revealed to me that it was she who had hurt her son, unable to bear his screams when he was, she now recognised, teething. She was so timid in daily life, and in her presentation with me, that this revelation was truly shocking, and hard to believe. Maja began to give voice to her anger, sense of displacement and revulsion at the way her partner treated her and flirted with other women, while constantly accusing her of sexual infidelity. Her own mother had been promiscuous and left her family when Maja was nine, leaving her largely in the care of her older sister. Her father had been depressed and hardworking, but not emotionally present for her.

When we first met, Maja told me that her main source of comfort was her son, whom she loved, but when he cried she found it unbearable, and described how his screams pierced her, and 'broke her'. Although she did not articulate this, it seemed clear to me that his cries resonated with her own internal distress, and traumatised her, leaving her feeling shaky and undone. She eventually told me that she had often handled him violently when he cried, and then felt guilty and scared by her own rage. On the day, she had broken his arm she had been on her own, after a violent argument with her partner, who had called her a whore and hit her. She had tried to call her sister but couldn't find her and felt totally alone and frantic. When her son had begun to scream she couldn't comfort him and said that as she looked at him she saw a reflection of her face. She repeatedly twisted his arm until she felt something snap and was then terrified by what she imagined she had done, calling her partner to explain how the baby had fallen, and going with them to the Emergency Department. This act of violence had brought about concern, help and protection for her son, but also, for herself. Her sense of guilt was profound and, I believe, predated rather than followed her assault on the baby.

Over the course of therapy, she disclosed not only her fantasies of harming her husband, but her own self-harm, and traced this to her hatred of her own body.

The link between her anger at the mother who abandoned her, her own body, signifying as it did her mother's and her husband, became clear, and she decided to leave him, after taking on a job where she made some friends and gained a sense of self-worth. She also took on a nursery place for her son, and found that was very helpful in reducing her wish to use him as a target onto which to displace her anger. Although this work was complex and delicate, her insight and engagement helped her to face the most unacceptable aspects of herself, and to trust herself to parent her vulnerable young son. Within the context of her toxic partnership with a violent, and often absent partner, she displaced her aggression onto her son, an unwitting participant in this destructive relationship. She appeared to use him as receptacle for her own feelings of helplessness and powerlessness, and ultimately as a signal to the outside world that she was locked in a vicious partnership.

## Medea crimes

Revenge through murder of children is the cruellest punishment that can be inflicted on the other parent, and on the children themselves; threatening to kill the children is one of the most powerful threats used to make a partner stay in an abusive relationship. Both men and women are capable of killing their own children in order to punish partners whom they feel have wronged them. When the perpetrators turn the murder weapon on themselves, they express a clear wish to die with their children and not to be held accountable for their murder.

In some cases, it appears that the loss of the relationship either precipitated or catalyzes depression, making homicide followed by suicide seem the only solution. The main motive in those cases is hopelessness and despair, rather than a straightforward wish for revenge, although it is well established in psychoanalytic theory (Hyatt Williams, 1998) that the suicidal impulse also contains within it a homicidal one. This can clearly be seen in the cases of women with whom I have worked, who have attempted to kill themselves along with their children, but have 'failed' to do so, although succeeded in murdering at least one of their children. They often describe a sense of deep regret that they are still alive, and feel that their task is incomplete.

Cases of attempted suicide, alongside murder, where the mother appears to have loved the children and attempted to 'take them with her', rather than wanting their deaths to be a form of vengeance may indicate maternal narcissism. In such a case, it is clear that the mother has not been able to conceive of her children's separate and discrete existence, continuing beyond her own life. Her profound inability to know where her body ends and her children's begin leads to these tragic consequences.

Despite the fact that children are most at risk of violence, including death, within their own families, 'stranger danger' is far easier for the public imagination to bear – it is much more palatable to locate sources of evil outside the home, in faceless 'others', than to look at the chilling reality of violence, sometimes fatal, that takes place in the domestic realm, perpetrated by family members. It is also simpler to place blame entirely on one parent and to locate savage impulses in him. However, it is often the case that, if one partner actively kills a child, the other has colluded with him (or her), by looking away. The accomplice parent may have been aware of their partner's murderous feelings, abusive behaviour and dangerous potential but turned a blind eye, or even facilitated the cover-up, perhaps providing an alibi or helping to hide the body of the victim – her own child. At the point where a child is killed they have become so objectified, so 'other' and non-human, that the disposal of the body is seen as a necessary part of the act. In a sense, it completes the annihilation of their existence that has already taken place.

## Self harm and self harm by proxy

Female violence often takes the form of self harm. The woman's own body can be understood to represent that of her mother, symbolically embodied in her own, and so she turns her violence against herself. This aggression serves both as re-enactment and revenge, creating an addictive and dangerous pattern of activity that replaces thought and prevents intimacy with another. At times the woman's choice of violent partner is also a form of 'self harm by proxy'. For some women, violence by their partners serves as a form of self harm, as they can hurt themselves brutally without using needles, knives, razors or matches on themselves. This rids them of unconscious guilt, fits a pattern that may have been modelled by their own mothers and further erodes any sense of their own self worth. Furthermore, it powerfully reinforces the notion that violent action is the most effective means for evacuating disturbing feelings. This resort to the world of bodily action, reaction and pain is familiar, and can even offer a form of bitter comfort. Physical pain is the conduit for intimate relating and the currency of communication. The contact made through violence is one that shatters the integrity of body boundaries and can leave scars and signs of this contact. It has a visibility and immediacy that is shocking to those who do not operate in this world of visceral contact, and also has sexual connotations and aspects that create their own disturbance and excitement. The symbolism of scarring, caused by self-inflicted wounds or those caused by others would be an important area of psychoanalytic research, drawing on the significance of the skin, as described by Esther Bick (1968) and more recently Ulnik (2007) and Lemma (2010).

## Technical considerations in the treatment of female perpetrators in violent relationships

The issue of avoiding a re-enactment of toxic coupling in the treatment with women who have committed acts of violence against their partners or children is central. It is easy to fall into a punitive or protective relationship with the patient in therapy, who can evoke strong feelings of anger or a powerful wish to rescue.

This can be understood as an unconscious projection by the patient of wishes to be either punished in accordance with her own guilt feelings, particularly awakened if she has left or 'abandoned' her violent partner, or to be rescued and transformed. The latter is the unconscious wish to be 'reborn' and to receive the protective and loving care of which they were deprived in early life, and that appeared to be met through the violent relationship that has now broken down.

Both powerful wishes can be projected directly and may resonate with the therapist's own unconscious needs and fantasies. The power of projective identification with these aspects of the patient and her history is intense, and offers a rich source of communicative data. The therapist may, at times, become identified with the controlling, punishing partner, who scolds the other for her perceived weakness and reluctance to leave destructive situations; she may feel frustrated and angry, using interpretations as form of violence. This may leave the patient feeling humiliated and battered. At other moments she may be in danger of enacting the role of the fantasised saviour, who offers endless succour and care. Acting into these wishes is ultimately unhelpful and will not allow the patient to find her own sense of containment and self-efficacy and to express and own the rage she feels. Rosenfeld (1987) describes the powerful force of such countertransference responses as resulting from the therapist's wish to perform 'a corrective emotional experience'. This urge must be resisted if the patient is to be helped, to articulate and process what has previously been unbearable. In the case of violent women, the sense of deprivation underlying their fury can invite an acting out of reparative wishes, coupled with a real fear of awakening their anger.

There is little sense of a shared sadness and joint participation in destruction within these partnerships but a much more dramatic quality in which one party is the victim and the other the perpetrator of violence. In Paula's case, she saw herself clearly as the aggressor and felt infuriated by her passive husband. She found it painful to acknowledge her own vulnerability. The splitting and rigidity of the roles can lead to a reductive understanding of the relationship that the therapist can act into, unconsciously falling into the role of the perpetrator or victim themselves. To help the woman entrenched in these dynamics, it is essential that she can be enabled to recognise the sense in which she has unconsciously allowed her partner to enact her violence for her, or, unleashed her own rage against her children, rather than simply submerging herself in a sense of despairing powerlessness. Enabling this recognition will not be possible if the therapist is judgemental or persecutory but can be assisted by the robust neutrality of a therapeutic stance. As in other cases of forensic psychotherapy treatment, the therapist acts as an auxiliary superego that is not cruel and relentless. The potential for sadomasochistic re-enactments within the therapy itself is significant and must be borne in mind.

There are other risks for the woman who allows this work to reach her. As she gains awareness of her own hostility, both towards her partner and her children, her defensive structure will be weakened and the resultant threats to her psychic integrity can generate increased self-harm or suicidal feelings. Her sense of guilt and beginnings of awareness of her own aggression can lead to a persecutory rather than reparative depression and the increased risk of self destructive action is important to monitor. Again, the containment and insight that can be offered within a strong therapeutic relationship can help the woman to survive the emergence of this persecutory guilt.

The link between homicidal and suicidal urges (Hyatt Williams, 1998; Motz, 2001/2008) is particularly strong in mothers who have fragile conceptions of themselves and narcissistic ways of relating to others. Their children are viewed as objects, reflecting aspects of themselves, including hated parts that they disavow. In the case of murderous couples, there is an unconscious contract between the two that enables acts of profound cruelty, deception and betrayal. This creates the conditions for child abuse and murder, as well as the killing of other third parties who pose a threat to the couple, or whose torture and death provide a form of excitement for them. Welldon (2012) describes situations in which children are deliberately killed by a couple as examples of 'malignant bonding'. A couple unites in their desire for cruel re-enactments, sometimes for sexual excitement, in which children are used as objects to be tortured and violated for the pleasure of adults. She explains how in some cases the children's suffering is recorded for the purpose of homemade pornography. The sadomasochism involved in such sexual torture can be seen as a form of rehearsal for the actual killing; the murder has happened time and time again in fantasy before it is enacted in real life.

This powerful link between homicidal and suicidal feelings is essential for the therapist to bear in mind as, when insight increases, so too does the wish to punish oneself. This insight can also be seen when a female accomplice to killing reclaims her projected aggression, and acknowledges her own murderousness. Once she is no longer able to locate these unacceptable and frightening states of her mind in her partner, her psychic equilibrium is jeopardised and suicidal feelings may then surface with catastrophic intensity. Just as a mother who has actually killed her own child, albeit in a psychotic state, may become seriously destabilised as the psychosis recedes and she recovers insight, so too can a woman who has configured herself as a passive, tragic victim in the murder become deeply depressed as she recognises her own active part in the crime. She has also killed off hope, as represented by her child, which may lead to profound helplessness and depression (Adshead, personal communication).

This process of insight is evident when child abusers, who have acted as part of a couple or a gang, begin to recognise the extent of their own individual culpability and cruelty. Through forensic psychoanalytic psychotherapy they can begin to acknowledge their own responsibility and finally give thought to the damage they have inflicted, neither of which will have occurred during their immersion in the abusive activity, and the partnership that fed on such sadism. A psychotherapeutic approach that recognises the painful, paradoxical juxtaposition of both victim and perpetrator in the same person is crucial. This will trace the individual pain and disturbed patterns of relating that is disguised within the complex and dangerous dance of the couple (Clulow, 2001; Welldon, 2009).

## Conclusion

When working with women who are entangled in violent and abusive relationships, it is essential to bear in mind that they too can be perpetrators within these toxic couples. The projection of aggressive impulses into the (male) other within these violent couples can serve to disguise the fact of female violence, but the sensitive practitioner needs to look below the surface and accept the fact of female perpetration in order to allow the woman to speak about her own unacceptable feelings and impulses, and engage her in the real work of therapy. The dual role of the woman as both victim and perpetrator in intimate partner violence can be replicated and re-enacted in the therapy as the therapist feels pulled into the role of victim or aggressor themselves. It is also essential to remain vigilant about the risk to any children in the household, as they can become the targets of the couple's shared rage, or the receptacle of the poisonous feelings of either partner. Working with individuals or with couples who are enmeshed in destructive dynamics requires acute awareness of the possibility of re-enactments in the therapy, and the need to resist these, and to remain still in the eye of the storm.

## Disclosure statement

No potential conflict of interest was reported by the author.

## Note

1. Details have been changed to protect confidentiality

## References

Adshead, G. (June 2013). Communication at joint presentation in Oxford at a conference on Philosophy and Psychiatry in the Consulting Room, organized by the International Association for Forensic Psychotherapy.

Bick, E. (1968). The experience of skin in early object relations. In M. Harris Williams, (1987) (Ed.), *Collected papers of Martha Harris and Esther Bick*. Perthshire: Clunie Press.

Clulow, C. (2001). Attachment, narcissism and the violent couple. In C. Clulow (Ed.), *Adult attachment and couple psychotherapy* (pp. 105–118). London: Routledge.

deMause, L. (1990). The history of child assault. *The Journal of Psychohistory*, *18*(1), 1–29.

Dutton, D. G., & Holtzworth-Munroe, A. (1997). The role of early trauma in males who assault their wives. In D. Cicceti & R. Toth (Eds.), *The Rochester symposium on development*. Rochester, NY: University of Rochester Press.

Dutton, D. G., & Nicholls, T. L. (2005). The gender paradigm in domestic violence research and theory: Part1 – the conflict of theory and data. *Aggression and Violent Behavior*, *10*, 680–714.

Freud, A. (1936). *The ego and the mechanisms of defense* (Vol. 2). New York: International Universities Press.
Freud, S. (1916). Criminals from a sense of guilt. *Standard Edition, 14*, 332–334.
Glasser, M. (1979). Some aspects of the role of aggression in the perversions. In I. Rosen (Ed.), *Sexual deviation* (2nd ed.). Oxford: Oxford University Press.
Hyatt Williams, A. (1998). *Cruelty, violence and murder*. London: Karnac.
Johnson, M. (2008). *A typology of domestic violence: Intimate terrorism, violent resistance, and situational couple violence* (Northeastern Series on Gender, Crime, and Law). Boston: Northeastern Press.
Lemma, A. (2010). *Under the skin: A psychoanalytic study of body modification*. London: Routledge.
Morgan, D. (2007). *Lectures on violence, perversion and delinquency*. London: Karnac.
Motz, A. (2014). *Toxic couples: The psychology of domestic violence*. Hove: Brunner Routledge.
Motz, A. (2001/2008). *The psychology of female violence: Crimes against the body* (2nd ed.). Hove: Brunner Routledge.
Rosenfeld, H. R. (1987). The influence of narcissism on the analyst's task. In *Impasse and interpretation*. London: Tavistock Publications Ltd. The New Library of Psychoanalysis.
Ulnik, J. (2007). *Skin in psychoanalysis*. London: Karnac.
Welldon, E. V. (1996). Introduction. In E. V. Welldon & C. van Velson (Eds.), *Forensic psychotherapy: A practical guide*. London: Jessica Kingsley Press.
Welldon, E. V. (1988). *Mother Madonna Whore: The idealisation and denigration of motherhood*. London: Free Association Books.
Welldon, E. V. (2009). Dancing with death reprinted. In *Playing with dynamite (2011)*. London: Karnac.
Welldon, E. V. (2002). *Ideas in psychoanalysis: Sadomasochism*. London: Karnac.
Welldon, E. V. (2012). The malignant bonding. In J. Adlam, A. Aiyegbusi, P. Kleinot, A. Motz, & C. Scanlon (Eds.), *Therapeutic milieu under fire*. London: Jessica Kingsley Press.

# 3 Man unlock: out of sight, out of mind

## Art psychotherapy with a woman with severe and dangerous personality disorder in prison

Jessica Collier

*Art Psychotherapies, Offender Care Services, Central and North West London NHS Foundation Trust, London, UK*

'3 Man Unlock' refers to the status of prisoners who are considered so volatile that they cannot be let out from behind their doors without three officers present at all times. This paper uses clinical material to illustrate the use of art psychotherapy to contain the trauma and violent acting out of a woman in a prison setting, whose status was frequently '3 Man Unlock'. The powerful projections from behind this locked door pervaded the landing, and it began to resemble the woman's mind: fragmented, split and paranoid. Through the development of a relationship with the art psychotherapist and the making of images, these toxic projections became part of a narrative that enabled the woman to express her feelings and see them contained, perhaps allaying the fear that her anxiety would overwhelm those around her and instigate a further lock-up. This woman's work illustrates the fear and dangerousness prisoners may feel themselves, and the cycles such punitive environments may re-enact.

## Introduction

Fear of attack is a constant part of the institutional dynamic in a forensic setting where the physical security of the actual building and the psychological security of a boundaried therapy session might be undermined by punitive or humiliating strategies used to relieve staff anxiety (Hinshelwood, 1993). Institutional and staff responses may stimulate unconscious re-enactments of abuse or trauma from the patient's past or of the trauma of committing the violent act itself (Hinshelwood, 2012; Ruszczynski, 2012; Scanlon, 2012).

In this paper, I aim to demonstrate that using image-making, within the containment of a therapeutic relationship, can help to make sense of conscious and unconscious communications, both in the work with the patient, in relationships with colleagues, within the institution itself, and ultimately in relation to society.

Using image-making to recognise primitive defences including splitting, projective identification and self-harm as wordless responses to the existence of trauma, both the act of violence perpetrated and the re-enactments of earlier traumas, can be acknowledged, witnessed and thought about. Unresolved trauma remains live in many of the women engaged in art psychotherapy in this environment and where this is psychologically active and likely to influence behaviour, in particular acting out rather than thinking (Bateman 1998; De Zulueta, 1998) this may lead to increased risk, which must be safely contained. Bracha Ettinger proposes in her work the idea of wit(h)nessing (Pollock, 2010, 2012). This is an aesthetic concept that brings together the notion of witnessing an individual's experience and feelings, while simultaneously being with them emotionally, of being present in their current telling of events. Art psychotherapy brings these psychoanalytical, creative and aesthetic ideas together.

I will consider more about unconscious communication and the way art psychotherapy can illuminate an individual's experience more closely in a detailed case study, which I hope will crystallise ideas based in art psychotherapy and attachment theory, object relations theory and in particular the concepts of projection and identification. I will connect this with the wider issues of the institutional transference and institution-wide projections and acting out.

## Art and psychotherapy

There is often a misunderstanding in clinical settings of the distinction between teaching arts and crafts and art psychotherapy (Waller, 1984). Throughout the prison, I am generally addressed by staff and prisoners as the art therapy teacher, the art and craft woman, the art lady or any number of permutations with the notable exception of art psychotherapist. Where the crossover does exist is in the possibility of art making meaning. Grayson Perry, a maker whose work confronts social issues including dysfunctional family relationships and child neglect, suggests that the desire to make art is innately human when he states '. . . I think there is a thing where the human being, the human mind has this amazing capacity to transform traumatic events . . . art is expressing one's universal wound, the wound of living a finite life of incomplete meanings' (Perry, 2013).

Given Grayson Perry made his name making pots, this might also be an opportunity to recognise Winnicott's concept of holding (Davis & Wallbridge, 1981) and Bion's concept of the container and contained (Bion, 1967) and the creative resonance these metaphors have in the thinking and practise of art psychotherapy (Dalley, 2000; Killick, 2000). Images contain meaning implicitly which may make not knowing and holding uncertainty more tolerable.

## The prison as container

To conceive of prison as an environment where art psychotherapy can take place, it is necessary to recognise its importance as a physically secure place for women who may live on the outside with the daily obstacles of addiction, mental health issues, violence, abuse and trauma. This primary acknowledgement of the importance of the physical container is paramount in offering the women the opportunity to use art psychotherapy where it may be unlikely their lifestyle outside would enable any consistent engagement (Adshead, 1997; Aulich, 1994).

In contrast to the chaos of living in the community, the prison regime and structure is centred on discipline, particularly ideas of reward and punishment known as incentives and earned privileges (IEPs). Women who behave well progress to enhanced landings where they are entitled to privileges including extra time unlocked. Women who are disruptive are put on 'basic' and lose privileges including their television or the right to associate with their peers. Violent or dangerous behaviour is met with transfer to the Care, Rehabilitation and Separation Unit (CRSU), colloquially referred to as the 'seg', where privileges are removed and the prisoner must sit an adjudication to decide how long she must spend segregated from less disruptive prisoners. Most women reside at ordinary location, and this accounts for the majority of the landings in the prison. There is a mixed group of women residing here who have committed a wide variety of offences and appear to cope reasonably well with the prison regime and the forced proximity to one another. There are separate landings for lifers and women who are detoxing from drugs or alcohol. In addition, there is a Healthcare Assessment Unit where women who are vulnerable or who are not coping can be monitored for transfer to hospital or supported to move back onto ordinary location.

This highly structured setting may be seen as physically containing and easily comprehensible. However, there exists the inevitable contradiction between prison's primary focus on security, punishment and discipline and art psychotherapy's primary focus on creative curiosity, reflection and understanding. This generates an inherently complex conflict. Furthermore, the staff and the prison setting itself, the brick mother, may reflect many of the problematic dynamics of the women's original families (Aiyegbusi & Tuck, 2008). Relationships between staff and the women can appear enmeshed or avoidant, and especially with those women who show personality disorder traits, which make up 50% of the female prison population (Jewkes, 2007) volatile and humiliating. There are regular splits where sides are taken or favourites preferred (Main, 1957) and important professional or peer relationships are frequently terminated abruptly, stimulating unresolved trauma around loss. The prison's security measures mean women are not told transfer dates and have no power to move around the prison to attend appointments. This provokes uncertainty that leads, paradoxically, to extremes of psychological insecurity, the foundation on which most of the violent offences by these women may be constructed. Thinking is commonly replaced by action, and women may respond to their distress through physical solutions. Distress in the female prison population, where the ability to regulate emotion is often limited, frequently manifests as violence, which in this context is primarily self-harm. This may momentarily act to sooth the woman's distress or give her some sense of control (Motz & Jones, 2009), but it equally offers the staff an opportunity to respond easily and concretely themselves. To use dressings or medication to offer physical relief, or to exercise a seemingly valid excuse to become angry or punitive, may be a welcome relief from the anxiety such behaviour engenders. In the meantime, the women's silent or mute psychological call may be overlooked. This violent acting out plays a part in the re-enactment of difficult and abusive relationships by the women, staff and the institution, and can be potentially highly destructive and dangerous (Norton & Dolan, 1995; Ruszczynski 2012; Scanlon & Adlam, 2012). It is essential to be cautious and acknowledge the toxic projections and acting out by both parties within the therapeutic relationship. An awareness of the discharging of unconscious projections and acting out using primitive defences including splitting, collusion and denial, by the therapist as well as the patient, is vital in understanding what is happening within the therapeutic process.

## Working in prison

I believe it is fundamental to understand the motivation I have for working in such a disturbing environment with such vulnerable individuals. Intellectually and politically, I can justify my motivation as an extension of my feminism. I believe that women have been ill treated by the criminal justice system and that historically education and learning in prison has been poor. Baroness Corsten reported that she found the women's estate '. . . sadly lacking in the concept of emotional literacy, the base from which all learning starts' (Corston, 2007, p. 7).

Underlying this, however, working with such primitive and violent emotions has forced me into uncomfortable realisations about my own life experience and emotional needs. This personal curiosity is essential. I believe that to be effective as an art psychotherapist I must be able to suffer when projections hurt and not just defend myself or counter-attack. It is as crucial to avoid emotional detachment as emotional over-involvement, and to do this safely, I must appreciate my own vulnerabilities and be aware of the difficult feelings and personal responses my patients may bring up in me (Temple, 1998; Yakeley & Adshead, 2013). If I do not recognise these feelings, then I am likely to unconsciously project them back on to my patients and colleagues just as my patients do to me. I must continually use supervision to assess my own internal conflicts and contradictions to work safely in what can feel like an unsafe situation. In addition, understanding counter-transferential responses is essential in discerning risk (Hinshelwood, 2012). For the women, art psychotherapy can reveal conflict, uncertainty and contradiction. But it can also hold intolerable emotions safely together in the images and within the therapeutic relationship to be thought about and processed in due course.

## Case study

I'd like to focus on one case to give a better understanding of the complexity and intensity in the ideas I have outlined. I have chosen this case because it was difficult emotionally and intellectually, both the relationship with the patient herself but also in relation to splits in the team, my own acting out and the institutional response to her emotional and physical violence. However, while seeking some understanding of the dynamics of this relationship, I also want to reiterate that not knowing and holding uncertainty for a patient is a real and important part of the work, particularly when the staff, the institution and the patient herself may be looking for concrete answers and explanations. Bion suggests that we must be able to tolerate mystery and our own ignorance (Bion, 1990) if we are to support our patients, and I see this as imperative.

I also want to emphasise how closely I attempt to monitor my counter-transference during art psychotherapy sessions. The feelings or identifications I perceive can inform risk assessment as well as offer what feels like an authentic involvement that may help me to recognise what is happening. Hyatt Williams suggests that the transference relationship between therapist and patient is '...crucial and in a very complex way it is THAT relationship that enables the contemporaneous situation to be understood and any danger signs recognised' (Hyatt-Williams, 1998, p. 160).

In the following case, I found that I felt forgotten and marginalised, vulnerable and exposed, or useless and hopeless, all of which might be thought about as projections originating from the patient, the staff, including me, and the prison itself. An awareness of these counter-transferential feelings also helps me identify any resonance that the patient's experiences or relationships may have with my own personal history, and thereby mitigate my feeling overwhelmed, confused or acting out in response or retaliation to what the patient brings up in me (Evans, 2007).

I want to thank this patient, whom I will call Tina, for allowing me to use this material.

## Initial meeting

At the time we met, Tina was in her mid-20s and had served 6 years of a life sentence with a tariff of over 20 years. She had been convicted along with two male co-defendants of the murder of another male who had died from stab wounds following an attack in the street.

Throughout her incarceration, Tina had been moved all over the prison estate, which mirrored her childhood experience of continually moving around children's homes. As a child, before her removal into local authority care, Tina had suffered neglect and inter-familiar child sexual abuse. This pattern of abuse by trusted adults and peers continued recurrently in the children's homes and foster care placements she entered (Adshead, 2004).

Following her conviction, Tina had been categorised as having a 'dangerous and severe personality disorder' (DSPD). The DSPD programme (Department of Health, 1999) was introduced in the UK in specialised intensive units in selected prisons and forensic hospitals in 2001 for the treatment of patients assessed as posing a significant risk of serious offending or harm to others and whose risk was linked to their personality disorder. Classification depended in part on a score of 30 + on the Psychopathy Checklist-Revised (Hare, 2003) and on the individual having a diagnosis of at least one further personality disorder in addition to antisocial personality disorder. DSPD was widely viewed as controversial primarily as it had no legal or medical basis and was interpreted as a political definition originating from the government consultation paper 'Managing dangerous people with severe personality disorder' (Department of Health, 1999). The programme has more recently been disbanded in favour of a reconfigured national strategy for managing high-risk personality-disordered offenders based on a 'whole systems pathway' across the criminal justice system and National Health Service (Joseph & Benefield, 2012).

The vast majority of individuals who fulfilled the criteria of DSPD were male. Perhaps in part as a consequence of this classification, Tina was seen as an unusually demanding and dangerous woman who in the past had taken hostages, made weapons and assaulted staff. She was a prolific self-harmer and was seen as difficult to contain. She approached me following a violent self-harming incident while staying on the healthcare assessment unit and asked me if she could have some art therapy as she felt this was her last chance and she 'had to do something'. I conferred with the team managing her care and agreed to see Tina for three assessment sessions.

## Assessment

Tina brought her diary to show me, and it was full of death, gore, abuse and violence. My immediate feelings were that she would reject art psychotherapy and it would not be enough to hold all the mess. Retrospectively, I thought this ambivalence on my part might be something of my own fear of working with her violence and rage. Tina made an image and spoke eloquently and metaphorically about her sketches. She said that she felt boxed in, could only smile on the outside and her heart was mangled up. While drawing, she disclosed sexual abuse, a violent rape and her mother's own imprisonment for murder caused by an arson attack when Tina was a young child. She protested her innocence of her own murder charge, but the cycle of trans-generational trauma seemed unambiguous.

Tina's images appeared sketchy, unconfident and diagrammatic, describing her feelings rather than embodying them (Schavarian, 1992). Tina draws a small empty box surrounded by blank paper (Figure 1), and on the other side, she draws a black square, a kind of void, which she then folds up. It feels defended and I wonder if this is mirroring my reluctance to think about what she has done or her closing off her thinking as a defence to protect her from the trauma of what happened. Either way, I'm aware that there's the possibility of my colluding with her denial of the murder and I seem to be cutting off my own feelings and capacity to think in order to survive my time with her. Motz suggests that the

Figure 1.

most insidious attack on thinking within the therapeutic relationship is the invitation to collude with the denial of what has happened (Motz, 2010).

## The beginning

Following the assessment, we agree to continue the sessions. Tina is back on ordinary location so is expected to do her therapy in a room on the landing. She tells me that she feels judged doing it here and wants to continue to come to the healthcare assessment unit. She tells me that she feels as if I can read her. I'm acutely aware of somehow being groomed by her, and I find myself agreeing to all her requests, which feels dangerous. While I might use this feeling as a way to assess the risk, I also want to keep in mind the fear we all feel when seeking something new or unknown and that Bion suggests is an important part of the therapist's work. He writes that '... when approaching the unconscious – that is, what we do not know, not what we do know – we, patient and analyst alike, are certain to be disturbed... In every consulting room there ought to be two rather frightened people: the patient and the psychoanalyst. If they are not, one wonders why they are bothering to find out what everyone knows' (Bion, 1990 p. 4).

During these initial sessions, Tina is saddened that the psychiatrist she trusted has now left and she speaks about a friend who killed himself, and she tells me she knows that I will leave her too. Tina speaks about both hating and loving her mother while drawing a very faint frame around the edge of the paper. She tells me she is not going to hurt me, and as we talk about the two of us in the room together, Tina paints this image of two trees leaning towards each other (Figure 2). She says that it is a place where she was happy once and I wonder if it's about us in the room together. The trees are not close and there is water between them but the birds seem to bridge the two together. I suggest this idea,

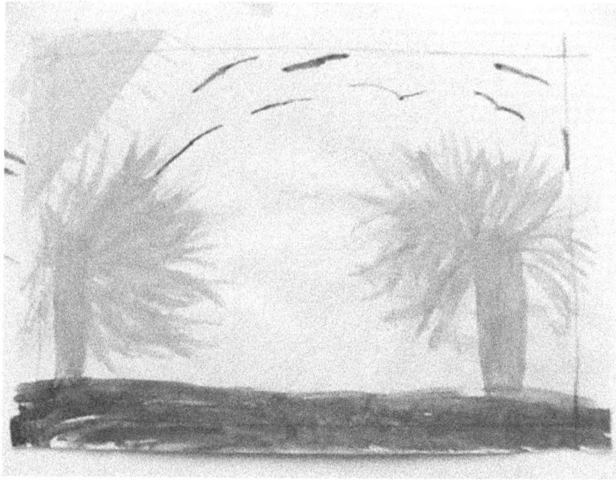

Figure 2.

perhaps prematurely, and Tina hides the image. This session feels difficult, but I feel myself beginning to engage and I wonder if Tina feels the same tentative relating?

By the end of the following session, my ambivalence has been usurped by sadness and I feel overwhelmed. She paints another frame, much heavier, and inside it makes a print. It sticks together, and she literally has to tear it apart leaving torn scraps of paper on both sides. It is damaged. She has been speaking about my gaze and tells a story about therapy in one of the children's homes where they covered her eyes and mouth if she didn't look at them or speak. Tina speaks about her experiences of neglect and abuse and how she thought as a child it was normal to be locked in a cellar. I think about the shame this must elicit and how my gaze might feel to her (Motz, 2010). Now Tina says she feels angry and she looks satisfied as she rips the paper apart. I think about her mother and about the separation she endured when she was imprisoned and how brutal it seemed when she pulled these two parts of the image away from each other. At the end of this session, Tina says 'all I want is a hug. I just want my mum to love me. I waited at the gates of children's homes for 9 years and she never came. I'm dogshit'.

Tina says she has been warned by another patient not to see me as I can 'read her thoughts'. I reply that I cannot read her thoughts or her images but I'm listening to her, and I'm reminded how these women have suffered so much emotional deprivation that being listened to may actually feel abusive and intrusive, responding to care as if it were abuse (Taylor, 2012). Tina again draws a frame and inside it a fragile, shaky, dry-looking pot plant under a small portion of sun. As she draws she describes the events leading up to the murder. She describes being beaten and kicked by her boyfriend who was also her pimp, and going out specifically to hurt someone so she could come to prison. This is the first time I think about Tina identifying with the aggressor at the point of the murder, re-enacting the abuse she had suffered for so long as a defence against her powerlessness and fragility. I think of Tina's despairing attempt to reduce her anxiety by changing from the passive victim to the active aggressor, assuming the attributes of her abusers to transform herself from the threatened to the threatening (Freud, 1936).

## Developing trust

Tina keeps coming to the sessions. We meet in the same room at exactly the same time each week. It is consistent. Tina is surprised she's still attending. She says 'you must be doing something right'. Outside of therapy she is being moved regularly around the prison from landing to landing.

Then, Tina is sent back to the 'seg' and has been told by staff that she is volatile and dangerous. She tells me she is not 'mad', so does not want to be on the healthcare assessment unit. I wonder if she is literally fighting for her sanity. She paints a thick black border while talking about how dangerous and violent her mother is and how her mother feels safe in prison because she knows if she's released she will kill again. I wonder if Tina is thinking about herself and feel momentarily frightened. I think of this fear as both a signal that I need to be aware of her potential violence but also a projection of Tina's own fear of the murderous part of herself. Tina has created a strong defensive box with several layers of walls (Figure 3), and I wonder if this is an internal prison, a place in which she can be safe. Tina finishes painting and tells me about a book she is reading. A teacher helps a child who has suffered abuse and gives her hope. I ask how and Tina replies, 'she is there for her and she listens'.

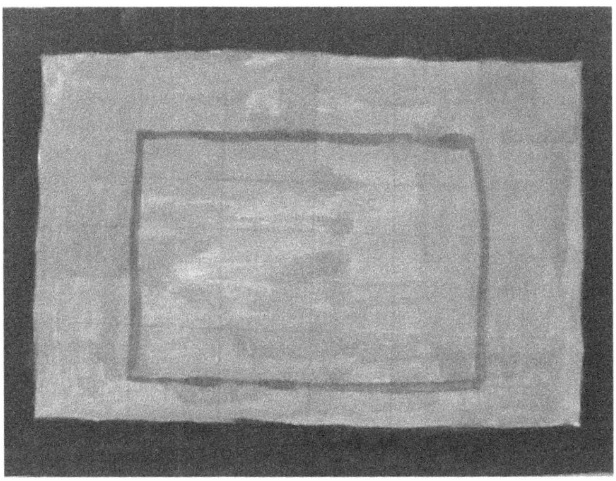

Figure 3.

## Attachment, idealisation and identification

Next time, Tina makes a lot more mess. She folds her image, but she does not tear it apart. It is stuck together and she leaves it stuck together. I think about how it has become *attached*. Tina asks how long I will see her for and asks if I will leave her too?

At this stage, it seems that Tina has begun to make an attachment to the therapist and the images. It's messy and I feel cautious. I'm also feeling anxious about the intensity of emotion and concerned that Tina is elevating me to a level where I can 'read' her in a way that no one else can. I'm worried about her splitting me off and idealising me, and how this might be acted out. Up to now the prison has been helpful in getting Tina to her sessions, and it has been agreed that a consistent therapy space will provide some continuity for her. But as the therapy progresses and Tina has been able to form an attachment, the prison itself appears less benign.

On arriving in the 'seg' to collect Tina for the next session, I am told by the landing governor that she will no longer be allowed to the health assessment unit and will have to have her sessions in the adjudication room. This is the room where sentences are passed down when a woman has broken prison rules. The governor is angry with Tina for her difficult behaviour. I protest vehemently and find myself in the security governor's office, head to head in what feels like my own adjudication. I seem to have taken on Tina's fighting stance and feel furious. I 'win' the argument but realise that my response is intense. I think of Tina's murderous rage and imagine how frightened she must have felt throughout her life and of how frightening she has become. I have to acknowledge my own primitive response to this dread. Perhaps this is my own defence mechanism, unconsciously identifying with Tina's aggression to protect myself from the fear and distress the work is instilling in me (Freud, 1936).

Tina arrives the following week and tells me she used to attack people who had a good life and once attacked a woman who looked like me. She tells me how physically strong she is while she draws a border and a square house. The house looks empty and barren (Figure 4). Tina doesn't want to look at it with me, and I think about her internal world and how empty and exposed she might feel.

When we meet again, Tina says 'I just have to tell you that if you never came back it wouldn't bother me, I wouldn't care' and she paints a single flower with a dry brush. She doesn't use water and paints straight from the tube. It is uncomfortable to watch and sounds and feels horrible, as if our being close is impossible to bear. I consider how overwhelming she might find our growing intimacy and how desolate she may find her own physical and emotional isolation (Glasser, 1979).

Throughout the next session, Tina asks me what I think the image she is painting is, as if she wants me to know (Figure 5). She tells me it has no meaning, it is just a mess and the flower should not be there. However, many weeks later, Tina tells me this is a depiction of the murder, which illustrates well how images can contain meaning when something is literally unsayable.

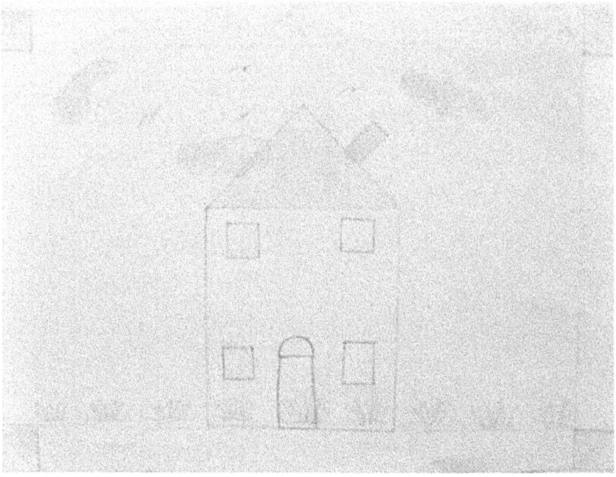

Figure 4.

## Shame, denigration and attacks on the therapy

In the week following this implicit but silent acknowledgement of her crime, Tina appears paranoid and dangerous. She shouts abuse at the officers and tells me she feels 'loose in her head'. I have to let her know that it doesn't feel safe to have a session. I wonder if Tina has broken an internal boundary in depicting this flower, her crime, and I feel conflicted and disloyal when I inform the team of my concerns about Tina's increased risk and mental well-being.

Tina has been taken back to the 'seg' and in this drawing she appears to have re-instated her own internal boundaries by locking herself up (Figure 6). She

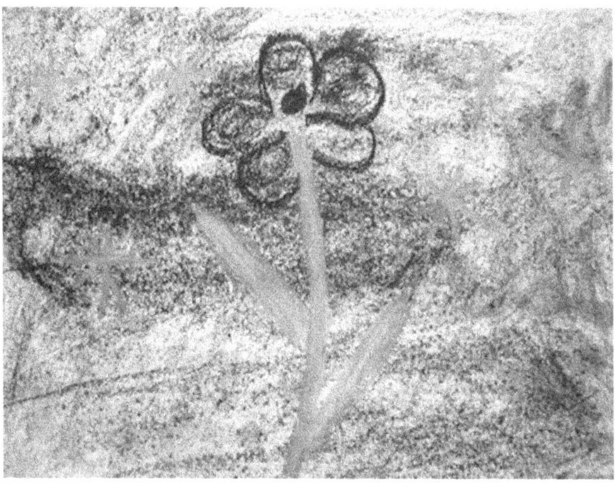

Figure 5.

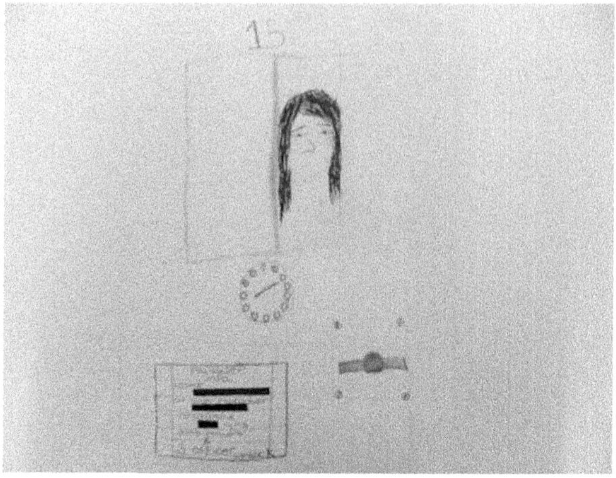

Figure 6.

seems to have re-enacted the entire narrative of her crime and punishment in this image and the previous flower image and her behaviour has mirrored this. She has mutely depicted the murder, broken down and been imprisoned. In addition, she has self-harmed and is refusing to eat. Tina says she feels weak and powerless and in the counter-transference this makes me feel very strong and safe. I wonder if I am enacting the institution's attitude to responding to violent crime. I feel paranoid, a parallel of society perhaps, impinged upon and invaded. I finish today's session by suggesting that next week we think about the precise number of sessions we should have. It seems as if I am even re-enacting the handing down of the sentence, perhaps as an unconscious paralleling of the offence and the institutional response (Scanlon, 2012).

Tina and I have agreed a framework to support her in applying for a prison-based therapeutic community for women with severe personality disorders. She is aware that they only accept women who admit their guilt in regard to their index offence. The work has felt intense, and I am aware of counter-transferential feelings of fear, paranoia, disappointment, rejection and anxiety. However, I also feel there is some hope being held in the therapy and in the relationship, which though at times feels idealised has not yet been completely denigrated. Then, Tina's closest friend dies unexpectedly in another prison, and she says she has 'more pain than the whole universe'. We do not talk but sit together with her image, which she folds over, saying she is ashamed of people seeing it.

The following week, I am told that Tina is too volatile to attend. I go to her cell to explain that I haven't forgotten her and that her session remains open. Tina shouts abuse at me through the hatch. I am shit, a liar, disgusting and she hopes I die of cancer or in a road traffic accident. She shouts that I just want her to talk about the murder. The verbal abuse continues even while I'm in the office. I feel tearful, shocked and misunderstood. I feel denigrated. Tina has done a remarkable job of letting me know how she feels and consequently I question my motivation to continue our work together. Hyatt Williams suggests that attacks on the process are inevitable. He wrote that the '... aim of the attacks, at least unconsciously, is to destroy the will to help, to abdicate from growing responsibility, and to drift back into a sense of aggrievement' (Hyatt-Williams, 1998 p. 261).

## Splitting and fragmentation

I have survived Tina's murderous projections but she is angry that I would think she would hurt me and she makes this image (Figure 7). As Tina draws the victim, she says *'yeauggh'* and appears disgusted. The mess is getting into her skin, under her nails and everywhere. In the image, a murder has happened. Tina does not fold or cover it up but hands it to me. She doesn't want to say anything about it. There is a planned break, and when we next meet, Tina has made a deep and dangerous cut in her leg and has smeared blood on her cell wall. It seems as if in the absence of a creative channel she has acted out the violence of the murder by assaulting her own body, or has perhaps attempted to annihilate her mental anguish by inflicting physical pain on herself. Ruszczynski proposes that individuals with no internal capacity to process anxieties, impulses or conflicts may use the external space they live in or their own bodies as a canvas to express their emotional states (Ruszczynski, 2012) and Tina seems to be doing exactly this.

She seems incapable of keeping herself safe and the staff team appear to be responding to Tina's powerful projections and seem scared. They begin to panic and are struggling themselves to keep Tina safe. Within the team action seems to have replaced thought and the prison is failing to contain the overwhelming

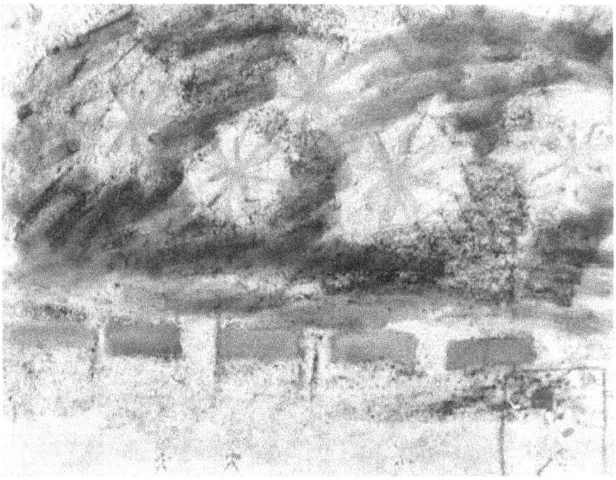

Figure 7.

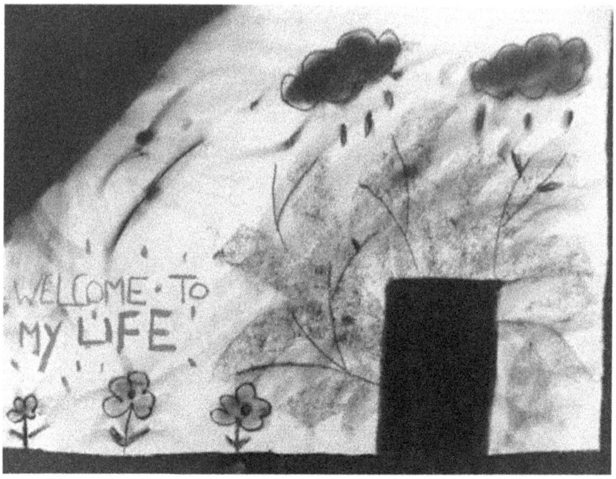


Figure 8.

anxiety Tina's embodiment of her trauma is creating. I find that a colleague has cancelled my session with Tina because he thinks it is dangerous. He has not consulted me and I feel furious, humiliated and anxious. I feel desperate for some hope in the next session but have to sit with the mess, the dust and the filth Tina's image generates. It is bleak and black and she folds it up and puts it aside.

During the next few weeks, I find I am unable to think and the sessions are constantly disrupted. It has been decided that Tina is to be transferred to a secure hospital. She is upset and is acting out violently. As a result, she is on and off '3 Man Unlock' and can only leave her cell for exercise if accompanied by three prison officers. Tina tells me her whole life she has been shut behind a locked door (Figure 8). She has said in a previous session, 'when they close my flap I am out of sight' and I think about the years of child sexual abuse she endured and the powerlessness the prison environment recreates by literally shutting her up.

Tina tells me she is scared of going to hospital as they will drug her so she cannot think. This fear seems to mirror my own and the team's inability to think as the levels of distress around her emotional disturbance becomes increasingly difficult to contain (Fonagy, 2004). Staff members are splitting now into those who feel supportive of Tina and have become over-involved and those who feel abused and worn down and have detached themselves. It feels as if her care is fragmenting and none of us can think (Aiyegbusi & Tuck, 2008).

There is uncertainty about Tina's transfer, and I remind her that we need to make definite plans for the final session. With this, Tina takes her work outside and rips it all up, screaming and crying out. I feel helpless and feel that nothing can be done. I take her empty folder to her and let her know she can put the work there, whatever condition it is in and I will continue to keep it safe. She cries that no one can help her, it is not possible, but when I return later in the day, her work is in her folder by my desk. It is in fragments (Figure 9).

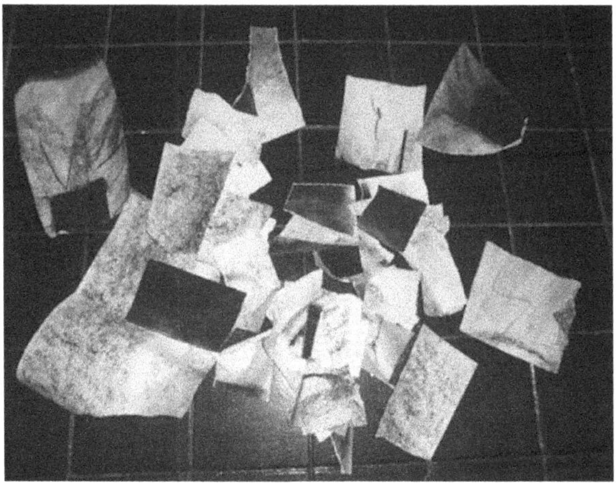

Figure 9.

## The ending

Tina makes her next image quietly but also wants to look at the 'murder' image again. She still doesn't want to talk about it. She labels today's image (Figure 10) 'before' and the murder image (Figure 7) 'after'.

Tina's referral to the secure hospital has been suddenly accepted, and she is told she could be transferred at any time. We agree that it will give her one definite ending to work with if we make the next session our last but Tina immediately walks out. I follow her and emphasise how important the ending will be. I tell her that throughout our work together I have felt hopeful, and Tina

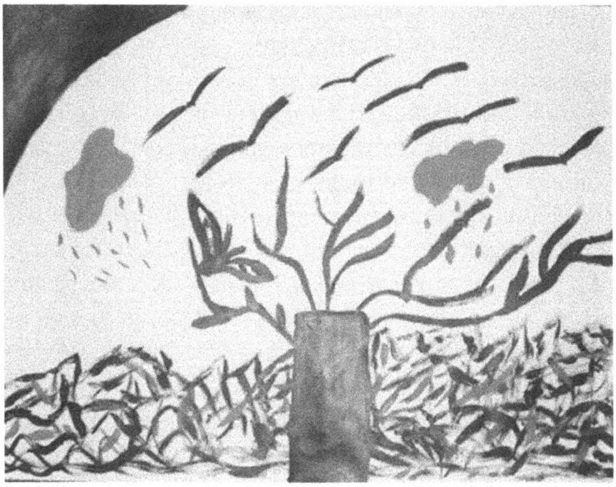

Figure 10.

begins to cry. We sit together quietly on a sofa in the healthcare assessment unit until the 50 mins is up and I encourage her once more to attend the final session.

The tree is alone in the water, and there is something on the horizon (Figure 11). Tina shows no emotion, but is able to stay almost to the end of the session. She gets up, but before she leaves she says to me, 'I appreciate you working with me. Most people are too scared to work with me, but you always stayed and weren't afraid'.

## Conclusion

My aim is that this case study emphasises the importance of what I believe art psychotherapy in prison can offer. Images can hold and contain difficult contradictory emotions, feelings and actions that cannot always be described verbally. The images themselves can be kept and looked after and the patient given time to begin to feel safe enough to think about them. This process can perhaps be thought about as a physical illustration of Bion's ideas around projective identification. Bion suggested the conceptual transformation of indigestible beta elements into metabolised alpha elements that occurs during alpha function resembled, and in many ways were identical to, the visual images with which we are familiar in dreams (Bion, 1967). There is something in the discharging of unprocessed feeling into images that allows them to be processed while in the therapist's care, before being brought out again for reflection as feelings that can be felt without becoming overwhelming. Tina was perhaps beginning this process of reflection in comparing her 'before' and 'after' images, but the suddenness of her transfer made further digestion impossible.

Tina had not only to contend with her own disintegrated inner world, but an institution that unconsciously repeated and compounded the rejection and loss she had been traumatised by, moving her around the estate from landing to landing and leaving her powerless. Tina's grief, following a sudden, unexpected and traumatic bereavement, created panic and was responded to by moving her suddenly to yet another institution. Her emotions became so overwhelming that it seemed none of us could think and the trans-generational failure to contain Tina's emotional disturbance, which led to her own violent offence, was re-enacted.

Tina wasn't able to speak much in the sessions, sometimes not at all. Often she would say nothing mattered or would get annoyed with me for sitting quietly. But her images gave her a voice and the consistency and boundaries of the therapy offered her a safe place where she could begin to look at her crime. She was able physically to describe what was happening for her, the mess, the fold of shame and the violence of her internal fragmentation.

This is what I would argue art psychotherapy is so good at. Images offer a different language, a language that can hold contradictions, nuances and physical acting out. These expressions of a patient's internal world can be put away, kept safe and brought out again when the patient is ready to start thinking.

I believe that art psychotherapy changes both the patient and the therapist. Working with Tina had a profound effect on me. It changed me and my hope and belief is that Tina was also able to internalise something important and permanent from our work together, something she could hold on to until she is ready to continue further. Tina moved to the hospital but she had, perhaps for the first time, experienced a relationship where she could be both creative and intimate with another person and with herself.

Peter Fonagy recognises the exceptional opportunity art making gives individuals to understand themselves when he states that 'art therapy invariably places the individual in relation to another – the creation of his or her imagination. There is something between the experiencing self and the self as a product of experience which is replicated in art therapy and may have much to teach us about... who we are' (Fonagy, 2012, p.90).

When I returned to prison after Tina's transfer, I was told that she had taken her art therapy images with her.

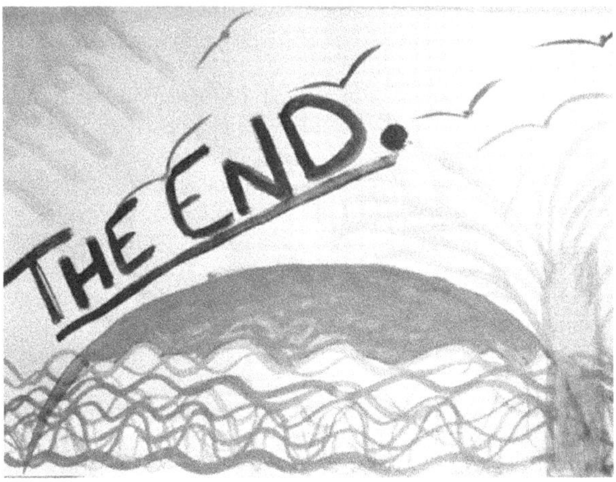


Figure 11.

## References

Adshead, G. (1997). The challenge of the victim. In H. Van Marle (Ed.), *Challenges in forensic psychotherapy*. London: JKP.

Adshead, G. (2004). Three degrees of security. In F. Pfafflin & G. Adshead (Eds.), *A matter of security*. London: JKP.

Aiyegbusi, A., & Tuck, G. (2008). Caring amid victims and perpetrators: Trauma and forensic mental health nursing. In J. Gordon & G. Kirtchuk (Eds.), *Psychic assaults and frightened clinicians*. London: Karnac.

Aulich, L. (1994). Fear and loathing. In M. Leibmann (Ed.), *Art therapy with offenders*. London: JKP.

Bateman, A. (1998). Defence mechanisms. In C. Cordess & M. Cox (Eds.), *Forensic psychotherapy: Crime, psychodynamics and the offender patient*. London: JKP.

Bion, W. R. (1967). *Second thoughts*. London: Karnac.
Bion, W. R. (1990). *Brazilian lectures*. London: Karnac.
Corston, J. (2007). Report executive summary. London: Ministry of Justice.
Dalley, T. (2000). Back to the future: Thinking about theoretical developments in art therapy. In G. McNeilly & A. Gilroy (Eds.), *The changing shape of art therapy: New developments in theory and practice*. London: Jessica Kingsley.
Davis, M., & Wallbridge, D. (1981). *Boundary & space*. London: Penguin.
De Zulueta, F. (1998). Theories of aggression and violence. In C. Cordess & M. Cox (Eds.), *Forensic psychotherapy: Crime, psychodynamics and the offender patient*. London: JKP.
Evans, M. (2007). Being driven mad: Towards understanding borderline and other disturbed states of mind through the use of the counter-transference. *Psychoanalytic Psychotherapy, 21*, 216–232.
Fonagy, P. (2004). The developmental roots of violence in the failure of mentalization. In F. Pfafflin & G. Adshead (Eds.), *A matter of security*. London: JKP.
Fonagy, P. (2012). Art therapy and personality disorder. *International Journal of Art Therapy: Inscape, 17*, 90.
Freud, A. (1936). *The ego and the mechanism of defence*. London: Hogarth Press.
Glasser, M. (1979). Some aspects of the role of aggression in the perversions. In I. Rosen (Ed.), *Sexual deviation*. Oxford: Oxford University Press.
Hare, R. D. (2003). *Manual for the revised psychopathy checklist* (2nd ed.). Toronto: Multi-Health Systems.
Hinshelwood, R. (2012). Personal trauma and collective disorder: The example of organizational psychodynamics in psychiatry in Hopper. In E. Hopper (Ed.), *Trauma and organizations*. London: Karnac.
Hinshelwood, R. (1993). Locked in a role: A psychotherapist within the social defence system of a prison. *The Journal for Forensic Psychiatry, 4*, 427–440.
Hyatt-Williams, A. (1998). *Cruelty, violence and murder*. Northvale, NJ: Jason Aronson.
Jewkes, Y. (2007). *Handbook on prisons*. Cullompton: Willan Publishing.
Joseph, N., & Benefield, N. (2012). A joint offender personality disorder pathway strategy: An outline summary. *Criminal Behaviour & Mental Health, 22*, 210–217.
Killick, K. (2000). The art room as container in analytical art psychotherapy with patients in psychotic states. In G. McNeilly & A. Gilroy (Eds.), *The changing shape of art therapy: New developments in theory and practice*. London: Jessica Kingsley.
Main, T. (1957). The ailment. *British Journal of Medical Psychology, 30*, 129–145.
Motz, A. (2010). *The psychology of female violence*. Hove: Routledge.
Motz, A., & Jones, H. (2009). The paradox of self-harm. In A. Motz (Ed.), *Managing self-harm: Psychological perspectives*. Hove: Routledge.
Norton, K., & Dolan, B. (1995). Acting out and the institutional response. *The Journal of Forensic Psychiatry, 6*, 317–332.
Perry, G. (2013, November 5). I found myself in the art world (Lecture 4). *Playing to the gallery*, [BBC Reith Lectures]. Platform Theatre, Central St Martins, London [Broadcast on BBC Radio 4].
Pollock, G. (2010). Aesthetic wit(h)nessing in the era of trauma. *EurAmerica, 40*, 829–886.
Pollock, G. (2012). After-affect? After image – trauma and aesthetic transformations, AHRC Research Fellowship Symposium, Anna Freud Centre, London.
Ruszczynski, S. (2012). What makes a setting secure? In J. Adlam, A. Aiyegbusi, P. Kleinot, A. Motz, & C. Scanlon (Eds.), *The therapeutic milieu under fire*. London: JKP.
Scanlon, C. (2012). The traumatised-organisation-in-the-mind. In J. Adlam, A. Aiyegbusi, P. Kleinot, A. Motz, & C. Scanlon (Eds.), *The therapeutic milieu under fire*. London: JKP.
Schavarien, J. (1992). *The revealing image*. London: Routledge.

Taylor, C. (2012). Complaints as a tool for bullying. In J. Adlam, A. Aiyegbusi, P. Kleinot, A. Motz, & C. Scanlon (Eds.), *The therapeutic milieu under fire*. London: JKP.

Temple, N. (1998). Transference and counter transference general and forensic aspects. In C. Cordess & M. Cox (Eds.), *Forensic psychotherapy: Crime, psychodynamics and the offender patient*. London: JKP.

Waller, D. (1984). A consideration of the similarities and differences between art teaching and art therapy. In T. Dalley (Ed.), *Art as therapy an introduction to the use of art as a therapeutic technique*. New York, NY: Routledge.

Yakeley, J., & Adshead, G. (2013). Locks, keys and security of mind: Psychodynamic approaches to forensic psychiatry. *The Journal of the American Academy of Psychiatry and the Law*, *41*, 38–45.

# The place of psychoanalytic psychotherapy in the treatment of high-risk personality-disordered offenders

Celia Taylor

*Millfields Unit, John Howard Centre, East London NHS Foundation Mental Health Trust, Hackney, London, UK*

Based on learning from the Dangerous and Severe Personality Disorder (DSPD) programme, the UK government is developing new services for the assessment and treatment of individuals with severe personality disorder who have committed serious offences such as murder, arson and rape. These offenders will largely be managed within the criminal justice system, with overall responsibility being taken by probation officers. Psychodynamic approaches have not been incorporated into these developments, apart from some supervision and reflective practice being offered to staff. This paper describes how one of the original medium secure DSPD units, based in the NHS, has adapted the psychoanalytic approach within its therapy programme. These adaptations are illustrated through a consideration of several patients who have committed parricide – the killing of a parent.

## Introduction

The public, and hence the media, has always had an uneasy relationship with those who commit serious crimes. On the one hand lies fascination: the entertainment is market saturated with violent films, games, detective novels and true crime analyses. On the other hand lies a deep-rooted dread of the stranger killer, rapist or child snatcher. Politicians are therefore not far behind, and many government strategies have been devised to address the circumstances of the latest notorious offence, in a vain attempt to ensure that it never happens again. Thus in the late 1990s, following a string of high-profile killings – most notably that of Lin and Megan Russell by Michael Stone in 1996 – the then Labour administration responded by planning changes to mental health legislation and a renewed focus on treatment. These were explicitly designed to prevent psychiatrists from 'washing their hands of dangerous psychopaths' (as the then

---

All patient details have been anonymised.

Home Secretary, Jack Straw, put it in 1998, after Stone's conviction), plug a large gap in services, and promote research into effective treatment. Thus in the early 2000s the 'Dangerous and Severe Personality Disorder' (DSPD) programme was born; it saw a large investment of money into the construction of four high secure units, two in hospitals and two in prisons, and three medium secure services, in what might well have been the most ambitious pilot of its kind. Within a few years, however, the programme was criticised on grounds of its low intensity, the failure of many of its offenders to progress and the lack of evidence of efficacy in reducing risk (Burns et al., 2011; Trebilcock & Weaver, 2010; Tyrer et al., 2007). The high secure hospital units in particular were deemed to be hugely costly, given their lack of positive results.

Following a consultation process, a revised approach took the learning from the DSPD programme in a different direction. The Offender Personality Disorder Strategy confirmed that high-risk personality-disordered offenders would from 2011 on be managed largely within the criminal justice system, and responsibility for overseeing sentence planning and progression along a defined 'pathway' would rest with the probation service (Joseph & Benefield, 2012). Input by specialist NHS clinicians would contribute to psychologically informed risk assessment and formulation, in order to guide management. Funds released from the closure of the DSPD unit in Broadmoor Hospital in 2012 were reallocated, both to prison-based 'Psychologically Informed Planned Environments' (PIPES; Bolger & Turner, 2013), specifically for inmates suffering from severe personality difficulties; and to supporting probation officers when these individuals were released into the community on licence. The strategy still allowed for transfer to hospital for assessment and treatment, but only in tiny numbers and when the offender's needs could not be met anywhere else. Quite how this provision would translate into individual, real cases was never defined.

These new pathways services are now well established. In London, a consortium of four mental health trusts (Oxleas; Barnet, Enfield and Haringey; East London; and South London and the Maudsley) called the London Pathways Partnership (LPP) gives largely psychological input to a progression unit in HMP Belmarsh; to an engagement and treatment unit in HMP Swaleside; to a young offenders' service in YOI Aylesbury; and to assisting probation officers across the capital (similar developments are taking place in the rest of the country). There is a small role for forensic psychiatrists where diagnosis and mental state are in question, and for a psychodynamic approach to supporting staff. The latter is provided by the Portman Clinic in the form of supervision and reflective practice. Despite the long history of psychoanalytic psychotherapy being used to treat people with problems arising from sexual or violent criminal behaviour, this approach has not been adopted within these projects beyond the use of certain concepts to aid understanding of acts that might otherwise be inexplicable. Indeed, psychoanalytic psychotherapy has been criticised for its 'lack of a standardized, structured intervention that can be applied with confidence'; for 'offering only theory'; and for 'lacking the empirical validation … that other treatment options provide' (Knabb, Welsh, & Graham-Howard, 2011, p. 127).

As Adshead points out (2001), great cynicism has been expressed as to the treatability of personality disorder, seemingly on the basis that it is not curable – a feature it shares with many other mental health problems, for example, schizophrenia. This article will describe one of the original medium secure DSPD services for high-risk personality-disordered offenders, within which the psychoanalytic approach has been used with measurable success, albeit in an adapted and integrated format. Fonagy, Roth, and Higgett (2005) have advocated such adaptations, as part of what they argue is a much-needed, fundamental change in the attitudes of psychoanalytic psychotherapists. In this they include 'ending the splendid isolation of psychoanalysis' (p. 677) through collaboration with different disciplines, and adaptations for those conditions that are especially hard to treat. The model described will illustrate how psychoanalytic thinking can inform thinking about, and responses to, the many challenges posed by this complex group, including their relationship to care, the importance of boundaries, the management of risk and the process of change itself. The article will particularly consider the characteristics, and progress in this form of therapy, of a number of men who have committed parricide – the killing of their fathers or mothers.

## A medium secure unit for personality-disordered offenders

From the outset, Millfields Unit incorporated psychoanalytic thinking and approaches to the treatment of this most demanding and complex group of patients. The service provides 16 beds for adult men who are deemed to pose a high risk of serious reoffending. Patients are transferred under the Mental Health Act (1983, amended, 2007), mostly from prison but some from high secure hospital; they have often been detained for years or even decades. Their offences include murder, rape, grievous bodily harm, arson, armed robbery and aggravated burglary. Those with predominantly paedophilic psychopathology are not accepted, in part because other services already exist for this group, but also because of the high prevalence of the severest forms of childhood sexual abuse among our men (Coid, 1992). Their personality difficulties are most commonly those of the antisocial and borderline kinds, but paranoid, narcissistic and avoidant features are not uncommon. To be offered a place the men must have a degree of motivation to engage in therapy (although varying degrees of ambivalence are both accepted and expected), and to possess some curiosity about their thoughts, feelings and behaviour. We have instituted a system of self-referral, which often sees the arrival of long, thoughtful petitions for consideration – prisoners being the last great letter writers of modern society.

By design, the programme is intensive and demanding, and patients stay for 2–3 years. The over-arching treatment model is that of a Therapeutic Community (TC). Central to the TC approach is the notion that the patients should be active participants in their own and each other's treatment, and that responsibility for the daily running of the community is shared among the patients and staff (Campling & Haigh, 1999). TCs consciously set out to establish a culture that fosters attachment by providing a secure base, provides containment through safe rules and boundaries, promotes communication and a common understanding, and includes everyone and everything that happens in the therapeutic task. The unit runs three community meetings and two small psychotherapy groups per week. The community meetings have a deceptively simple structure and purpose: a chair and vice chair are periodically elected by the whole community, and take responsibility for running and minuting the meeting. A set of ground rules, agreed and written down by the patients, is read out at the start. There is open disclosure of index offences when introducing new patients, staff or visitors. Designated patients give feedback on all group and individual therapy sessions, to ensure there are no secrets within the unit.

After this, the floor is open to discuss any difficulties – especially those that manifest themselves as breaches of boundaries, interpersonal aggression or exploitation – that are happening in the 'here and now': all such behaviour is seen as meaningful. This is the 'culture of inquiry' referred to by Tom Main (1946). The meeting provides a forum for exploring actions that have hitherto been used defensively to fend off thoughts and feelings. Commonly, unconscious transference patterns or conscious strategies stemming from childhood are played out in unwarranted hostility towards a particular individual – or, in the case of social workers for example, towards a group of people regarded bitterly as having failed to rescue them from abuse in childhood. The meeting is also a vehicle for patients and staff to exert their influence upon individuals whose attitudes and behaviour are upsetting to others or threaten their well-being. A 'senior resident' can have, by virtue of him having been through the same journey, far more credibility than the professionals – who tend to be seen as authority figures and therefore as untrustworthy. Griffiths and Hinshelwood (1997) have likened this to 'a form of psychodynamically-informed action learning' (p. 12) in which inquiry, thought and understanding take the place of violent deeds.

The small psychotherapy groups represent another psychoanalytic space, adapted in that, for example, group members and facilitators live and work together outside of therapy times. The small group model uses elements of group analytic psychotherapy, in particular thinking about the group as a complex unconscious network of interactions between individuals, subgroups and the whole group (Foulkes, 1975). As described by Montgomery (2002, p. 38), 'this can be understood as the shared ground of the group, which fosters a strong sense of belonging based upon the discovery, over time, of common experiences, difficulties and insights'. The aim of the groups is to reach an understanding of the patients' attitudes and behaviours and their unconscious underpinnings, which have led to the development of dysfunctional defence mechanisms and behaviours, including offending. Nevertheless, at times the facilitators have to think of ways they can draw attention to matters that are being avoided, minimised or justified. As in all groups, there will be resistance to the group process that is anti-therapeutic; with these patients, however, this is likely to take the form of delinquency and acting out. In order to keep the groups safe, the facilitators carry radios and wear alarms, while an extra member of staff remains nearby at all times. This is a further example of how the psychoanalytic approach, which generally assumes safety as a necessary pre-condition for treatment (McWilliams, 2004), must be adapted for those who have committed serious violence in the past, and might still.

Integrated within this framework of community meetings and small groups are additional, specific treatments that are deliberately eclectic, in order to meet the different and sometimes very individual needs of the patients. They include 9-month, weekly cognitive–behavioural groups addressing substance misuse and violent offending, art psychotherapy and individual psychotherapy. Each patient is also supported to develop a personal narrative or formulation that can give meaning to what has usually been a fragmented existence. We have found the variety of theoretical approaches to work well in combination, with some individuals needing to learn basic skills in emotional recognition and management before they can use the less structured small groups. Together, these therapies form a safe, reliable and confidential space that knits together theory and practice in a way that both patients and staff can understand (Bateman & Tyrer 2004). We work hard to preserve the day-to-day structure in the face of encroachments, because of its centrality in providing a holding environment (Gabbard, 1992) for seriously disturbed individuals: over time, even they come to miss their small group during therapy breaks. Adler (1982) has reflected that locked environments can provide a useful level of containment – similar to Winnicott's (1960) notion of a holding environment. Griffiths and Hinshelwood (1997, p. 1) have described the patient as creating a 'hospital in the mind that mirrors his inner world'. For offenders with severe personality disorder, this is likely to be an environment in which care givers can be expected to let them down at best, and behave sadistically at worst; this is the starting point for treatment.

Intensive exploration of the patients' offences would be demoralising if we did not also give them opportunities to succeed; indeed, some have never had such an experience before. We, therefore, place great emphasis on developing each individual's talents and strengths, as well as a sense of responsibility for self and others. Patients go through a formal application and interview process for paid unit jobs, such as magazine editor or shop worker. They can also be employed in our catering social enterprise, fulfilling orders for refreshments at staff training events or when we have visitors to the unit. Work is so important because it introduces a socially beneficial and creative means of sublimating aggressive or destructive energies (Menninger, 1942), and provides – in the right circumstances – a realm in which camaraderie, pride and a sense of being valued can be experienced. The need to work together also teaches tolerance of difference, and a healthy capacity to depend on others. These skills are much needed upon release into the community, where life is far less protected and untoward events can shake resolve.

In a surprising, but humbling, development, we have seen our former patients gather together to form their own social network – even to the extent of holding a 'small group' (as they continue to call their gatherings) in someone's living room when mutual support is particularly needed.

## Parricide

A number of men convicted of parricide – the killing of a parent – have been admitted to the unit. Parricide is an unusual offence involving less than 4% of all the UK homicides (Smith et al., 2010). It has been referred to as 'the schizophrenic crime,' (Clark, 1993), because it accounts for 20–30% of homicides committed by psychotic individuals (Marleau, Millaud & Auclair, 2003). However, more recent studies, of juvenile offenders especially, highlight the central significance of perpetrators having endured severe, long-term childhood abuse (Heide, 1994; Myers & Vo, 2012). This can be so harsh that it has been described as tantamount to torture by Mones (1994), who argues that 'battered child syndrome' should be considered as a legitimate defence in court. The sequelae of childhood abuse, which have been described as 'complex post-traumatic stress disorder' (Herman, 1992), include poor emotional control, depersonalisation and dissociation, difficulties with intimacy and identity confusion. Equally pernicious is the accompanying loss of a sense of agency and meaning in life (Livesley, 2003).

In a study of 10 men who killed their fathers (patricide), Singhal and Dutta (1990) found that many had a 'cruel and unusual relationships' (p. 43) with their victims, in that these fathers had been more punitive and shaming in comparison to a control group; the mothers, on the other hand, were more overinvolved and tolerant. Just before the killing, both sons and fathers tended to have been drinking alcohol, and were frequently involved in an argument. Another study found that just after the killing, sons are filled with a sense of relief and freedom, as opposed to remorse (Cravens et al., 1985). Freud (1900, 1905) believed the Oedipus complex to be the source of a wish that is present in all males to kill the father, thereby gaining possession of the mother. However, he viewed any tendency for this wish to reach consciousness as very different from more normal aggressive impulses. West and Feldsher (2010) helpfully added a Family Systems Theory understanding of the crime: common contextual features include the sons' isolation from external influences, demands from one parent for loyalty or to be rescued, an entrenched pattern of family battles and denial of the gravity of the family's difficulties. Weapons are often used in a context where the long-term suppression of rage and hatred leads to a 'pressure cooker' effect: a culmination of parental abuse that can no longer be tolerated.

Sons who killed their mothers (matricide) have reported seeing themselves as weak, inadequate, hopeless, dependent, confused about their sexual identity and unable to adopt a separate, adult male role; most still lived at home (Singhal & Dutta, 1992). Mothers were generally domineering, humiliating, possessive and sexually provocative, while fathers were passive or absent. In the early 1940s,

Wertham (1941) proposed an alternative to Freud's Oedipus complex to explain the crime of matricide. He conducted a psychoanalytic study of sons who had killed their mothers, which he published in a book called '*A Dark Legend*'. He suggested the existence in these men of an 'Orestes complex', choosing the name from Homer's story in which Orestes avenged his father's death by killing his mother and her lover Aegisthus. Wertham found that the sons generally had no prior history of delinquency, were excessively attached to their mothers, and often committed the murder in her bedroom following a trivial argument. The use of excessive force – so-called overkill – has also been recognised to be a frequent feature (West & Feldsher, 2010). While Freud believed that matricide is a displacement defence against incestuous longings, Wertham postulated that these men nurse a combination of sexual desire for, and hatred of, their mothers and ultimately transform fantasy about the killing into action.

## Application of the Millfields model to the crime of parricide

Almost every new patient experiences a severe kind of culture shock upon being transferred to the unit: prison involves long hours of 'bang-up', an often hostile-dependent relationship with officers, and the working assumption that (literal) attack might happen at any time. Preserving a macho stance is vital in an institution where weakness – especially of the emotional kind – is despised and exploited. When preparing an information pack for newcomers, some of our patients wrote, 'This is a chance to break the cycle – a place where people are civilised. There is no culture of criminality compared to prison'. The expectation is that new patients will start attending the community meetings immediately, and that they will disclose their offence. This is a particularly fraught time for the perpetrator of a parricide, which in our experience is a crime associated with the deepest levels of shame: this is because, at both an individual and a societal level, it violates two basic moral injunctions, namely that prohibiting murder, and that requiring parents to be honoured (Hillbrand et al., 1999). Such severe shame greatly elevates the risk of suicide, making residential treatment the only safe option. Usually, these men share only that they have been convicted of murder, and delay telling the whole truth for many weeks or months. Matricide is an especially difficult crime to 'own', given the idealisation by most offenders of their own mothers (often in the face of reality), and by society of mothers in general (Welldon, 1992). Curiously, it is not one of the crimes that are universally despised in prisons, unlike child sexual offences and violence to the very old or very young.

Within weeks, certain patterns of behaving and interacting becomes evident. Thus one matricide offender, Alex, presented as anxious to please, almost overobedient and highly conscientious. He rapidly engaged in all the available activities, and was almost unique in his failure to push boundaries. In community meetings, however, he was more than usually able to speak frankly and independently – except about his index offence – to his more delinquent peers.

His relationship with his brothers was understandably fractured, but from meetings with an elderly aunt a picture emerged of an almost 'Jekyll and Hyde' mother, whom Alex felt it had been his duty always to honour and obey. She had a terrifying temper, such that even her friends were scared of her, and exerted control over her sons by methods such as, leaving them outside the house all night and tying them to a drainpipe. Alex's memories were more focused on her charm and vivacity; she was 'great company' for him. Alex described his father rather contemptuously as having 'given up' and left the home long ago; apparently his very first comment on hearing of his son's offence was that he had felt like killing his ex-wife himself. After some months, however, we saw evidence of Alex's dysfunctional ways of managing his anger. At times, he would flare up briefly in irritation, only to quash the feeling and brood. During a planned meeting with his (female) education tutor, his (male) primary nurse – who was to support Alex with his work between classes – hurried into the room, having been slightly delayed. Alex angrily misperceived this as indicating the nurse's belief that he posed a risk to women (a sensitivity left over from his trial), but fumed over this in silence for a fortnight before being able even to mention it.

A hugely comforting therapeutic factor of the small groups is that of 'universality' (Yalom, 2005); the possibility of sharing human distress and receiving validation. In the case of a crime as rare as matricide, however, this is virtually impossible outside a highly specialist service. For the first time in a lengthy sentence that will span a decade, Alex had the chance to share with his small group how he killed his mother in an explosion of rage and violence that seemed to come from nowhere. Indeed, so out of character did he feel his actions to be, that he lives in fear of a future loss of control, and what he might potentially do. At the time, he had his mother had been disagreeing over his untidiness. Alex seemed to be an example of Megargee's subgroup of violent offenders who, unable to express their anger normally, eventually 'explode' and release all their rage and aggression at once, often in response to a seemingly trivial provocation (1966). While exploring the possible sources of Alex's extreme emotion, another parricide offender shocked him profoundly by pointing out some of his mother's evidently difficult behaviour – thereby giving Alex permission to think what had previously been unthinkable in relation to her. It is difficult to convey his sense of shock at the unconscious and forbidden thought becoming conscious and permissable, and his growing awareness thereafter of the extent to which he had capitulated to his mother's will in the name of loyalty and devotion.

A much younger matricide perpetrator, Scott, was by contrast confiding and gregarious from the day he arrived; this could be understood as the indiscriminate friendliness associated with inconsistency in caregiving (Pears et al., 2010). However, his precipitous talk soon began to disturb others, because of the way he spilled out his story in public areas – including at the dinner table, not sparing us the details of how his mother's decomposing body smelled. There was a repetitive, unprocessed feel to these confessions, as if they were being made for the very first time. Scott had been the victim from a young age of sexual abuse by his mother, who also forced him to watch horror movies that left him paralysed with terror. After being taken into care, he perfected his technique in distraction burglaries of elderly women who would, unsuspecting in the face of his polite and respectful manner, invite him into their home. The murder took place after he had gone back to live at home when he left care at 16 – 'because you only have one mother' – upon which the sexual abuse resumed, along with humiliating intrusions into his privacy, even in the bathroom. Unusually Scott had a co-defendant, a boy who had also been sexually abused and on whose behalf he could finally allow himself to feel a murderous rage. Scott very quickly recreated his role of protector within the unit, by initiating a potentially serious act of violence on the part of a volatile fellow patient around his own age. Two older peers stepped in to protect a nurse who was trying to hold a boundary about bedtime, resulting in one of them getting hit. Actual acts of violence are vanishingly rare in the unit, so this one led to much discussion in the community meeting on the following day. Feedback to Scott from his peers included the following comment about the true nature of his honourable (as he saw it) defence of his friend's 'human right' to stay up all night: 'You're trying to be good *to* each other, but you're not good *for* each other'.

Paul, a man of 25 years of age, committed patricide at the age of 19 years, during a blazing row in which intervened to prevent his younger sister from being hit by their father. In a dissociated, raging state, which he later could hardly remember, he bludgeoned his father to death with a dumbbell. The siblings then hid the body in the basement behind some old furniture and appliances. Paul went on to commit repeated armed robberies, at least sometimes (as he later admitted) to get himself detained once more in prison. From the age of 3 years, he had been forced to eat from a dog's bowl in the garden, and was frequently beaten and then shut in a cupboard as a punishment for his misdemeanours. Childhood experiences of extreme physical and emotional sadism are so common as to be almost a hallmark of severe personality disturbance. Reddemann and Sachsse (2000, p. 559) have pointed out that 'frequent, repeated, longish-duration, humiliating bodily mistreatment is aetiologically the most important factor in social dysfunction and the development of antisocial personality disturbance' (cited by Hoffmann & Kluttig, 2006, p. 14).

Such experiences as Paul's also fundamentally alter the individual's concept of, and relationship to, care. Thus he developed an intensely negative transference reaction to his primary nurse Jack, whose behaviour towards him he perceived to be cruel, unfair and humiliating, no matter how hard Jack tried to prove his professionalism and commitment. Hinshelwood (2002) has described the three central features of severe personality disorder as being suspiciousness towards help; internalisation of the original abuse as later self-abuse – Paul had a history of self-harming by punching his face black and blue – and internalisation of (and later identification with) an abusing figure, so the patient is then driven to abuse others, physically or psychologically. Thus the provision of care within institutions can 'degenerate into an inhumane culture based on condemnation, control and a reverberating bitterness' (Hinshelwood, 2002, p. S25). This tendency, which Moore (2012) has called 'the pull to punish', is from time to time expressed by staff in the unit in demands for severe 'consequences' for patients' actions to be imposed, which are in reality little more than sanctions. History has shown that these patients do not respond to punishment, which all have experienced on many occasions; the goal instead is to introduce a consequence that involves thinking about their impact upon others. Both our Staff Support and Reflective Practice Groups have occasionally seen staff express hatred for a patient, usually – and understandably – when they have been singled out for particular venom. Staff need a great deal of support, as well as safe opportunities to process both hostile and seductive projections, if severe splitting and the adoption of extreme positions are to be avoided (Main, 1957).

The 'living learning' environment of the TC (Jones, 1952), together with the intensive psychoanalytic and other therapies our patients undertake, afford them frequent opportunities for 'corrective emotional experiences' (Alexander & French, 1946, p. 66) and for the internalisation of more benign relationships with others. Over time, and with much repetition, Paul gradually re-experienced his need to protect others, but with the new possibility of a non-violent resolution in that the cruelty and rejection he anticipated – and at times nearly brought about through his highly threatening behaviour – were not forthcoming. As the Alexander and French (1946) point out, this requires a shift away from traditional therapist neutrality, towards a much more active expression of humane compassion, empathy and encouragement. In a TC all staff must join this endeavour to provide a benign environment, in which safe boundaries are nevertheless clearly and effectively maintained (Hoffmann & Kluttig, 2006).

## Making a difference

In these days of evidence-based medicine, and of the emphasis on 'what works', conducting research into the efficacy of an expensive treatment approach is necessary both on ethical grounds and for survival. A recent evaluation of the service therefore set out to examine the effectiveness of the treatment model, based on clinical monitoring and outcome data collected annually throughout each patient's stay (Wilson et al., 2014). Two violence risk measures, the Historical-Clinical-Risk 20-item scale (HCR-20; Douglas et al., 2013), and the Violence Risk Scale (VRS; Wong & Gordon, 1999–2003) were rated over a 3-year period, based on observations and clinical impressions of behaviour within the TC, engagement with treatment and activity undertaken with the purpose of reducing risk (e.g. preparation of leave plans or arrangement for support after discharge). Each patient's Responsible Clinician rated whether patients had been successfully discharged or not. Self-reported symptoms were also monitored, using the Symptom Checklist 90–Revised (SCL90-R; Derogatis, 1994). This provides an indication of nine point-in-time symptom dimensions (somatisation, obsessive–compulsive, interpersonal sensitivity, depression, anxiety, hostility, phobic anxiety, paranoid ideation and psychoticism), and three global indices of distress (Global Severity Index [GSI], positive symptom distress index and positive symptom total). Analysis was performed on an 'intention-to-treat' basis in which, if the patient was discharged (successfully or unsuccessfully) before the 3-year mark, the final available value of the assessment was carried forward and used as a proxy for 3-year outcomes.

The results showed evidence of decreasing risk and psychological symptoms as patients progressed with treatment. VRS dynamic scores showed consistent statistically significant decreases each year from initial assessment, whilst SCL90-R GSI scores significantly decreased from initial assessment to the third year of treatment. The significant reduction in patients' psychological distress suggests that the therapy provided successfully alleviates the anxiety and arousal that have so much potential to exacerbate the risk of future violence, and complicate rehabilitation. Analysis of HCR-20 scores was not conclusive, with an initial improvement over 2 years leading to an increase in risk in the third year. This result may coincide with some patients commencing community leave in the later stages of treatment, which necessitates a change in scoring the HCR-20 outside the secure and contained environment of the unit and into a context that by its very nature contains a multitude of unknown variables and therapeutic risks for patients. A further study is now planned, to conduct an in-depth, qualitative analysis of patients' experiences of the treatment, which it is hoped will have more to say about the important subjective, interpersonal and creative aspects of therapy.

## Conclusions

This evident double standard highlighted by Adshead (2001), in which the bar for successful treatment of personality disorder is set so much higher than for other conditions, seems to reflect an ongoing ambivalence on the part of all but a few clinicians, commissioners, politicians and members of society about providing services for a group that is still widely despised and repudiated (Lewis & Appleby, 1988). It is to be hoped that a combination of therapeutic enthusiasm, compassion and use of the knowledge-base of psychoanalysis to generate innovative treatment approaches (Fonagy, Roth & Higgett, 2005) will allow the new generation of services for this neglected group to survive and prosper. To this list might be added: good evidence of effectiveness, since a goal that all can agree to be worthwhile is the successful prevention of further deaths, including of the mothers and fathers of such afflicted children.

## Disclosure statement

No potential conflict of interest was reported by the author.

## References

Adshead, G. (2001). Murmurs of discontent: Treatment and treatability of personality disorder. *Advances in Psychiatric Treatment, 7*, 407–415. doi:10.1192/apt.7.6.407

Adler, G. (1982). Recent psychoanalytic contributions to the understanding and treatment of criminal behaviour. *International Journal of Offender Therapy and Comparative Criminology, 26*, 281–287. doi:10.1177/0306624X8202600311

Alexander, F., & French, T. (1946). *Psychoanalytic therapy: Principles and applications.* New York, NY: Ronald Press.

Bateman, A., & Tyrer, P. (2004). Services for personality disorder: Organisation for inclusion. *Advances in Psychiatric Treatment, 10*, 425–433. doi:10.1192/apt.10.6.425

Bolger, L., & Turner, K. (2013). *Psychologically informed planned environments: Model description document V1.0.* London: National Offender Management Service & NHS England.

Burns, T., Yiend, J., Fahy, T., Fazel, S., Fitzpatrick, R., Sinclair, J., ... The IDEA Group. (2011). Inclusion for DSPD: Evaluating assessment and treatment (IDEA) (March 2006–August 2009). Final Report to NHS National R&D Programme on Forensic Mental Health.

Campling, P., & Haigh, R. (1999). *Therapeutic communities: Past, present and future.* London: Jessica Kingsley.

Clark, S. A. (1993). Matricide: The schizophrenic crime? *Medicine Science and the Law, 33*, 325–328.

Coid, J. (1992). DSM-III diagnoses in criminal psychopaths; the way forward. *Criminal Behaviour and Mental Health, 2*, 78–95.

Cravens, J. M., Campion, J., Rotholc, A., et al. (1985). A study of 10 men charged with patricide. *American Journal of Psychiatry, 142*, 1089–1092. doi:10.1176/ajp.142.9.1089

Derogatis, L. R. (1994). *Symptom checklist 90–R: Administration, scoring, and procedures manual* (3rd ed.). Minneapolis, MN: National Computer Systems.

Douglas, K. S., Hart, S. D., Webster, C. D., & Belfrage, H. (2013). *HCR-20 (Version 3): Assessing risk of violence: User guide.* Burnaby: Mental Health, Law, and Policy Institute, Simon Fraser University.

Fonagy, P., Roth, A., & Higgitt, A. (2005). Psychodynamic psychotherapies: Evidence-based practice and clinical wisdom. *Bulletin of the Menninger Clinic, 69*(1), 1–58. doi:10.1521/bumc.69.1.1.62267

Foulkes, S. H. (1975). *Group analytic psychotherapy, method and principles.* London: Gordon & Breach.

Freud, S. (1900). The interpretation of dreams. In J. Strachey (Ed.), *The standard edition of the complete psychological works of Sigmund Freud* (Vol. IV, pp. ix–627). London: Hogarth Press.

Freud, S. (1905). Three essays on the theory of sexuality. In J. Strachey (Ed.), *The standard edition of the complete psychological works of Sigmund Freud* (Vol. VII, pp. 123–246). London: Hogarth Press.

Gabbard, G. O. (1992). The therapeutic relationship in psychiatric hospital treatment. *Bulletin of the Meninger Clinic, 56*, 4–19.

Griffiths, P., & Hinshelwood, R. D. (1997). Actions speak louder than words. In P. Griffiths & P. Pringle (Eds.), *Cassel hospital monograph no. 1: Psychosocial practice within a residential setting.* London: Karnac.

Heide, K. M. (1994). Evidence of child maltreatment among adolescent parricide offenders. *International Journal of Offender Therapy and Comparative Criminology, 38*, 151–162. doi:10.1177/0306624X9403800207

Herman, J. (1992). *Trauma and recovery.* New York, NY: Basic Books.

Hillbrand, M., Alexandre, J. W., Young, J. L., & Spitz, R. T. (1999). Parricides: Characteristics of offenders and victims, legal factors, and treatment issues. *Aggression and Violent Behavior, 4*, 179–190. doi:10.1016/S1359-1789(97)00056-6

Hinshelwood, R. D. (2002). Abusive help – helping abuse: The psychodynamic impact of severe personality disorder on caring institutions. *Criminal Behaviour and Mental Health, 12*, S20–S30. doi:10.1002/cbm.2200120604

Hoffmann, K., & Kluttig, T. (2006). Special section: Psychoanalytic and group-analytic perspectives in forensic psychotherapy. *Group Analysis, 39*, 9–23. doi:10.1177/0533316406062321

Jones, M. (1952). *Social psychiatry: A study of therapeutic communities*. London: Tavistock.

Joseph, N., & Benefield, N. (2012). A joint offender personality disorder pathway strategy: An outline summary. *Criminal Behaviour and Mental Health, 22*, 210–217. doi:10.1002/cbm.1835

Knabb, J., Welsh, R. K., & Graham-Howard, M. L. (2011). Treatment alternatives for mentally disordered offenders: A literature review. *Psychology, 2*, 122–131. doi:10.4236/psych.2011.22020

Lewis, G., & Appleby, L. (1988). Personality disorder: The patients psychiatrists dislike. *British Journal of Psychiatry, 153*, 44–49. doi:10.1192/bjp.153.1.44

Livesley, W. (2003). *Practical management of personality disorder*. New York, NY: The Guilford Press.

Main, T. (1946). The hospital as a therapeutic institution. *Bulletin of the Menninger Clinic, 10*, 66–70.

Main, T. (1957). The ailment. *British Journal of Medical Psychology, 30*, 129–145. doi:10.1111/j.2044-8341.1957.tb01193.x

Marleau, J. D., Millaud, F., & Auclair, N. (2003). A comparison of parricide and attempted parricide: A study of 39 psychotic adults. *International Journal of Law and Psychiatry, 26*, 269–279. doi:10.1016/S0160-2527(03)00037-2

McWilliams. (2004). *Psychoanalytic psychotherapy: A practitioner's guide*. New York, NY: The Guilford Press.

Megargee, E. (1966). Undercontrolled and overcontrolled personality types in extreme antisocial aggression. *Psychological Monographs, 80*, 1–29. doi:10.1037/h0093894

Menninger, K. A. (1942). Work as a sublimation. *Bulletin of the Menninger Clinic, 6*, 170–182.

Mones, P. (1994). Battered child syndrome: Understanding parricide. *Trial, 30*, 24–29.

Montgomery, C. (2002). Role of dynamic group therapy in psychiatry. *Advances in Psychiatric Treatment, 8*, 34–41. doi:10.1192/apt.8.1.34

Moore, E. (2012). Personality disorder: Its impact on staff and the role of supervision. *Advances in Psychiatric Treatment, 18*, 44–55. doi:10.1192/apt.bp.107.004754

Myers, W. C., & Vo, E. J. (2012). Adolescent parricide and psychopathy. *International Journal of Offender Therapy and Comparative Criminology, 56*, 715–729. doi:10.1177/0306624X11410587

Pears, K. C., Bruce, J. J., Fisher, P. A., & Kim, H. K. (2010). Indiscriminate friendliness in maltreated foster children. *Child Maltreatment, 15*, 64–75. doi:10.1177/1077559509337891

Reddemann, L., & Sachsse, U. (2000). Traumazentrierte Psychotherapie der chronifizierten, komplexen Posttraumatischen Belastungsstorung'. In O. F. Kernberg, B. Dulz, & U. Sachsse (Eds.), *Handbuch der Borderline Storungen* (pp. 555–571). Stuttgart/New York, NY: Schattauer.

Singhal, S., & Dutta, A. (1990). Who commits patricide? *Acta Psychiatrica Scandinavica, 82*, 40–43. doi:10.1111/j.1600-0447.1990.tb01352.x

Singhal, S., & Dutta, A. (1992). Who commits matricide? *Medicine Science & the Law*, *32*, 213–217.

Smith, K., Flatley, J., Coleman, K., Osborne, S., Kaiza, P., & Roe, S. (2010). *Homicides, firearm offences and intimate violence 2008/09. Supplementary volume 2 to crime in England and Wales 2008/09* (3rd ed.). London: Home Office.

Trebilcock, J., & Weaver, T. (2010). Multi-method evaluation of the management, organisation and staffing (MEMOS) in high security treatment services for people with dangerous and severe personality disorder (DSPD). Report written on behalf of the MEMOS study team.

Tyrer, P., Barrett, B., Byford, S., Cooper, S., Crawford, M., Cicchetti, D., … Seivewright, H. (2007). *Evaluation of the assessment procedure at two pilot sites in the DSPD programme (IMPALOX Study)*. London: Ministry of Justice.

Welldon, E. V. (1992). *Mother, madonna, whore: The idealization and denigration of motherhood*. London: Karnac books.

Wertham, F. (1941). *A dark legend: A study in murder*. New York, NY: Sloan and Pearce.

West, S. G., & Feldsher, M. (2010). Parricide: Characteristics of sons and daughters who kill their parents. *Current Psychiatry*, *9*, 20–38.

Wilson, K., Freestone, M., Taylor, F., Blazey, F., & Hardman, C. (2014). Effectiveness of modified therapeutic community treatment within a medium-secure service for personality-disordered offenders. *Journal of Forensic Psychiatry & Psychology*, *25*, 243–261. doi:10.1080/14789949.2014.908317

Winnicott, D. W. (1960). The theory of the parent-infant relationship. *International Journal of Psychoanalysis*, *41*, 585–595.

Wong, S. C. P, & Gordon, A. (1999–2003). *Violence risk scale*. Saskatoon: Department of Psychology, University of Saskatchewan.

Yalom, I. D. (2005). *The theory and practice of group psychotherapy* (5th ed.). New York, NY: Basic Books.

# 'This is the pain I feel!' Projection and emotional pain in the nurse–patient relationship with people diagnosed with personality disorders in forensic and specialist personality disorder services: findings from a mixed methods study

Anne Aiyegbusi[a] and Daniel Kelly[b]

[a]*West London Mental Health NHS Trust, Southall, Middlesex, UK;*
[b]*Director of Research/RCN Chair of Nursing Research, School of Healthcare Sciences, College of Biomedical and Life Sciences, Cardiff University, Cardiff, UK*

This paper reports the lived experience of the nurse–patient relationship in specialist forensic and therapeutic community (TC) settings for people diagnosed with personality disorders (PDs), from the perspectives of both nurses and patients. A sequential mixed methods study incorporating quantitative Delphi study data with qualitative insights based in the tradition of phenomenology and underpinned by a psychoanalytic paradigm. Purposive samples of nurses and patients currently involved in providing or receiving the nurse–patient relationship in TC or forensic mental health settings were included. Qualitative data analysis resulted in three main themes identified by nurses and patients regarding their experiences of the nurse–patient relationship. They were: (1) Pain: processing or passing on? (2) System of social defences. (3) What helps? This paper focuses on the first 'pain: processing or passing on' of the three themes. This theme describes highly painful emotional phenomena arising primarily from patients' traumatic antecedents, suffusing interpersonal transactions, including the nurse – patient relationship. This is reported as experienced by nurse and patient participants. The findings emphasise the relevance of integrating Bion's theory of psychological containment and Bowlby's attachment theory into the nurse–patient relationship in services for people diagnosed with PDs.

## Introduction

People diagnosed with personality disorders (PDs) have long presented a challenge to nurses within in-patient settings. The main therapeutic tool of mental health nursing is the nurse–patient relationship and this has not always been experienced as effective in the face of the tremendous negative, emotional impact and risk behaviours that are associated with patients diagnosed with PDs. In turn, patients diagnosed with PDs have described their experiences of in-patient mental health care as dissatisfying and invalidating, even re-creating early traumatic experiences. A sequential mixed methods study integrating theoretical frameworks derived from phenomenology and psychoanalysis is reported. The study aimed to provide an understanding of the nurse–patient relationship with people diagnosed with PDs in forensic and specialist in-patient settings from the perspective of those with lived experience. That is, nurses and patients. One theme from the findings of the study offers a potential explanation for the painful experiences that both nurses and patients report within the nurse–patient relationship and associated interactions. It is hypothesised that enduring and raw emotional pain emanating from patients' unprocessed traumatic antecedents becomes activated during in-patient care and is projected onto and sometimes into nurses with the use of risk behaviours providing extra purchase. One function of this unconscious process is for the patient to communicate their emotional distress in the context of an environment that is actually or perceived to be unresponsive.

Nurses working in some of the services included in this study were able to work positively and therapeutically with the challenging and complex phenomena, employing interpersonal approaches informed by Bion's theory of psychological containment and Bowlby's attachment theory. It is suggested that this approach may offer an effective way for nurses to understand the aspects of PD patients' presentations that nurses have traditionally found difficult and also, provide a compassionate approach to supporting their recovery within in-patient settings.

## Personality disorders

PDs have been described by the American Psychiatric Association (APA, 2013) as pervasive patterns of cognition, affect, interpersonal behaviour and impulsivity that lead to distress on the part of the sufferer, their environment and/or those with whom the sufferer has relationships. Ten distinct types of PDs described in the *DSM V* (APA, 2013) are grouped into three clusters; A, B and C. Cluster B PDs are most likely to be experienced by people who use mental health and forensic services (National Institute for Mental Health in England [NIMHE], 2003). Cluster B PDs are particularly associated with behaving harmfully to self and others and consist of borderline, histrionic, narcissistic and antisocial PDs, which are also sometimes referred to as severe PDs. Borderline PD is the most extensively researched of the PDs (NIMHE, 2003).

Though not a criterion for diagnosis within the *DSM V*, the development of severe PDs is associated strongly in the literature with early experiences of trauma (Herman, 1992, Herman & van der Kolk, 1987). Psychological trauma and neglect that occur within an attachment context can impact on a person's developmental trajectory to a degree that results in the emergence of PDs (Adshead, 1998; Fonagy & Bateman, 2007).

## Literature review

### *The perspective of people diagnosed with PDs*

People diagnosed with PDs have described their mental health conditions in terms of disorders of attachment (NIMHE, 2003) and sequelae of early traumatic experience (Castillo 2003). Ramon, Castillo, and Morant (2001) found that 88% of sample of people diagnosed with PDs who had used mental health services, reported histories of physical or sexual abuse. Of those, 80% had experienced trauma during their childhoods. Ramon et al. (2001) question whether PD diagnoses actually serve to mask the real problems, including ongoing symptoms of trauma.

When the in-patient experience of people diagnosed with PDs has been captured within the research literature, their interactions with professionals, including nurses are often described as negative and hurtful (Fallon, 2003; Ramon et al., 2001; Rogers & Dunne, 2011). A diagnosis of PD has been associated with stigma, activating prejudice and negative attitudes on the part of staff (Fallon, 2003; Rogers & Dunne, 2011). Castillo (2003) suggests that experiences of early trauma in the lives of people with PD get re-enacted during their contact with mental health services.

### *The nursing perspective on PDs*

The published evidence focusing on the nurse–patient relationship with people diagnosed with PDs suggests that nurses in acute and forensic in-patient settings struggle to work therapeutically with this client group. Difficulties appear to be located in the characteristic ways that people diagnosed with PD behave during interpersonal transactions with health care professionals. These behaviours are described by nurses as self-harming, manipulative, emotionally blackmailing, bullying, intimidating, suicidal, threatening, violent and rule-breaking (Bowers, 2002; Richman, 1998; Woollaston & Hixenbaugh, 2008). Nurses have reported that they do not like to work with PD patients (Bowers, 2002; Richman, 1998; Woollaston & Hixenbaugh, 2008), finding them more difficult and less amenable to nursing interventions than are people diagnosed with other mental health conditions (James & Cowman, 2007; Markham, 2003; Markham & Trower, 2003). Murphy and McVey (2003) concluded that PD work is more demanding of nurses than is the case in any other field of mental health nursing.

In attempting to support the core nursing task of providing a relationship which is in and of itself therapeutic and capable of providing a holding and healing experience (Peplau, 1952; Stockwell, 1972) with people diagnosed with PDs, it may be important to understand what is happening within the interpersonal context that makes this so difficult to achieve. Through literature reviews, Bland, Tudor, and Whitehouse (2007) and Murphy and McVey (2003) suggest some PD patients experience emotional dysregulation and have unstable relationship styles that leave nurses feeling overwhelmed by negative affect. Emotional dysregulation involves the activation of multiple affects simultaneously, leaving the person overwhelmed and struggling to regulate their feelings or retain a coherent sense of themselves in relation to others (Linehan, 1993, Fonagy & Bateman, 2007). Importantly, dysregulation interferes with the person's capacity to accurately attribute intentionality to others' behaviours or motives (Fonagy & Bateman, 2007). This experience underpins unstable relationship styles and can have the effect on the patient of rapidly switching attitudes towards people (Bland et al., 2007). For example, nurses characteristically experience themselves to be idealised initially by the PD patient and then during an episode of dysregulated emotion this can abruptly change into intense denigration and accusation (Bland et al., 2007). The tendency towards either idealisation or denigratation of members of the team has been associated with splitting nurses into such polarised categories as 'good' and 'bad' (Bland et al., 2007, Woollaston & Hixenbaugh, 2008) and has been identified as a key source of conflict within teams that PD patients are perceived to cause (Woollaston & Hixenbaugh, 2008). A further example of unstable relationship styles could be witnessed in the way PD patients engage in attempts to avoid abandonment, which may be manifest in a need for prolonged interpersonal input from nurses. This is inevitably perceived by nurses to be to the detriment of other patients on the ward (Bland et al., 2007, Woollaston & Hixenbaugh, 2008).

Overwhelmed by the impact of negative affect generated during interpersonal interactions with PD patients, nurses have been observed to react in ways that are invalidating and disconfirming of the patients' underlying distress. Fraser and Gallop (1993) found that during interpersonal interactions with PD patients, nurses were less validating of their subjective experiences when compared with patients diagnosed with other mental health conditions. PD patients also elicit the most negative feelings and least empathy, or sympathy, from nurses when compared with patients who have other mental health diagnoses (Fraser & Gallop, 1993; Markham & Trower, 2003). Markham (2003) also found that nurses described more negative attitudes and perceptions about patients diagnosed with PD. Mason, Hall, Caulfield, and Melling (2010) found that nurses working in forensic services were more likely to perceive PDs as requiring behaviour management than treatment for a clinical condition. The picture to emerge from existing literature about interpersonal interactions within the nurse–patient relationship in forensic and acute mental health in-patient settings suggests that nurses commonly experience themselves as actual or potential victims of PD patients (Bowers, 2002; Woollaston & Hixenbaugh, 2008).

### *The relevance of a psychoanalytic approach*

Bowers (2002) sought to identify what supported positive nursing attitudes towards patients with PDs in high secure psychiatric services. He identified that nurses who understood the patients' challenging behaviours in terms of developmental manifestations of early traumatic experience, had more positive attitudes. In terms of employing a psychoanalytic approach to clinical practice, a number of authors have asserted its value for helping nurses to be aware of, and organise their therapeutic relationships with patients who, like those diagnosed with PDs, have adverse developmental histories including traumatic attachment experiences and abuse (Cremin, Lemmer, & Davison, 1995; Gallop & O'Brien, 2003; McAndrew & Warne, 2005). These recommendations are based on the type of interpersonal experiences that people with traumatic histories may unconsciously seek to recreate within the nurse–patient relationship (Bray 1999; Cremin et al., 1995; Evans & Franks, 1997; Jones, 2005). It is suggested that through unconscious processes of projection and projective identification, patients may apply interpersonal pressure on nurses to engage in relationships which re-enact their painful experiences with earlier intimates (Cremin et al., 1995). Paradoxically, what appears on the surface to be wilful destruction on the part of patients may, at an unconscious level, be a desperate but unfortunately, all too frequently fruitless attempt to communicate their need for psychological understanding and support (Cremin et al., 1995).

By providing a clear developmental model and a paradigm for elucidating unconscious interpersonal processes, a psychoanalytic approach to the nurse–patient relationship with people diagnosed with PD, may normalise otherwise confounding emotional and interpersonal phenomena and also provide a framework for informing effective relational nursing practice (O'Kelly, 1998; Warne & McAndrew, 2007; Winship, 1998). Importantly, a psychoanalytic framework may offer a model for working effectively with the parallel subjective conviction of being locked in role as a victim of the abusive other, which both personality disordered patients and nurses have reportedly experienced within the context of the nurse–patient relationship and associated interactions (Bowers, 2002; Castillo, 2003; Rogers & Dunne, 2011; Woollaston & Hixenbaugh, 2008).

## Methodology

### *Aims of the research*

The research aims that are relevant to the findings reported in this paper are:

- Establish primary nurses' experiences of the nurse–patient relationship with people who have PDs in therapeutic community (TC) and secure mental health settings.
- Establish people diagnosed with PDs' experiences of the nurse–patient relationship in TC and secure mental health settings.

### *Research design*

This was a sequential mixed method study, integrating quantitative Delphi study data with qualitative insights, based in the tradition of phenomenology, and underpinned by a psychoanalytic paradigm.

### *Services included in this study*

The services included in this study were all specialist mental health services for the care and treatment of people diagnosed with PDs. A brief description of each service is provided here.

### *Therapeutic community*

The residential, psychoanalytic TC provides treatment for informal patients suffering from severe PDs. Treatment consists of a combination of individual psychotherapy and psychosocial nursing. Length of treatment is typically for 12 months. As part of the TC model, patients are actively involved in the care and treatment of each other, including through the daily running of the services.

### *Dangerous and severe personality disorder*

Patients admitted to dangerous and severe personality disorder (DSPD) services are at very high risk of causing serious harm to other people, are often admitted as they approach the end of a lengthy custodial sentence, having been convicted of severe violent or sexual offences. Criteria for admission are explicitly stated and include diagnoses of severe PDs including high psychopathy scores as measured by the revised psychopathy checklist (PCL-R: Hare, 1991, 2003). Additonally, PD and risk must be functionally linked meaning that risk of serious harm to others is directly attributable to PD. The UK government set up a series of pilot services which aimed to effectively assess and treat this population who had previously confounded mainstream high security hospital treatment programmes, including by undermining security procedures (Department of Health, 1999; Department of Health, Home Office and HM Prison Service, 2004). Two DSPD pilot services were developed in high security psychiatric hospitals. Following a review of the effectiveness of the pilots, a phased decommissioning programme has been implemented, with the strategic intention of re-investing resources from the DSPD pilots, to develop offender PD treatment pathways within the criminal justice system (Department of Health and National Offender Management Service, 2011).

### *Women's enhanced medium secure services*

Women's enhanced medium secure services (WEMSS) was conceived through the English national women's mental health strategy (Department of Health, 2002, 2003). A review that took place as part of the national strategy identified that women detained in high secure settings typically experienced complex mental health problems and presented challenging behaviours on a day-to-day basis within the setting. Nevertheless, they were considered to have been inappropriately detained within higher conditions of physical security than was required for the risk presented to the public. As a result, a new type of secure service was piloted which aimed to be gender sensitive and address the complexity of the patients' clinical needs, primarily through therapeutic relationships. Three WEMSS pilot services opened in England in 2007.

### *Sampling*

Purposive sampling was used throughout the study as the aim of the research was to gain an in-depth understanding of a unique experience, the features of which would only be known by the people who had lived that experience (Silverman, 2000).

### *Inclusion criteria*

The Delphi technique is a consensus method of research that typically seeks to establish expert consensus in a subject where no expert consensus currently exists (Goodman, 1987). In this study, an expert nursing consensus was sought with regard to the key clinical processes and practices for managing the nurse–patient relationship with people diagnosed with PDs. Participants had considerable experience, qualifications and clinical skills in the field of PD services.

For the qualitative interviews, participants were registered nurses who were currently working as a primary nurse within PD services.

For the qualitative focus groups, inclusion criterion was that all patients residing in the clinical services participating in this study could be included as long as their responsible clinician agreed that they had capacity to consent to do so.

### *Delphi*

Twelve nurses ranging from primary nurses to consultant nurses from three clinical sites participated in the Delphi. Participants were anonymous of each other. The first round of the Delphi consisted of participants providing their expert judgement about what the key nursing processes and practices for managing the nurse–patient relationship with people diagnosed with PDs are. The judgement of the participants was used to produce a questionnaire, which was then circulated to all the participants who rated how important each item was. The rated items were then circulated again and participants asked to rerate in the light of the overall panel ratings. Consensus was reached after three rounds.

Consensual Delphi findings were used to inform topic guides for qualitative methods. Details of Dephi findings, interview and focus group guides are available from the first author.

### *Qualitative interviews*

A purposive sample of 13 primary nurses from the three specialist services participated in in-depth qualitative interviews. By 13 interviews, no new themes were emerging. Therefore, it was judged that data saturation had occurred. As a result, no further interviews were conducted.

In-depth interviews were conducted in meeting rooms within the clinical services and were recorded and later transcribed verbatim.

### *Focus groups*

Twelve in-patients diagnosed with PDs participated in three focus groups.

Focus groups were conducted in clinical rooms within the services and were recorded and transcribed verbatim. The researcher was supported by a Practice Development Nurse during the focus groups.

### *Analysis of qualitative data*

Framework analysis was employed. Framework was developed in the 1980s at the National Centre for Social Research (Ritchie & Spencer, 1994). The term 'framework' is taken from the 'thematic framework' which is the central component of the method (Ritchie, Spencer, & O'Connor, 2003). This approach was underpinned further by theoretical principles outlined below.

### *Theoretical approach*

A hybrid theoretical approach was taken, integrating principles from Husserlian phenomenology and psychoanalysis. Husserlian phenomenology is concerned exclusively with the essence of conscious experience from the perspective of the person whose experience it is (Husserl, 1900/1970). Because of the possible association between unconscious processes and the difficulties experienced by nurses and PD patients during therapeutic relating (Bland et al., 2007; Bray, 1999; Cremin et al. 1995), a psychoanalytic perspective was also integrated by either facilitating participants' descriptions of unconscious processes or inferring them from participants' reports of emotional experience and behavioural responses.

### *Ethical approval*

A favourable ethical opinion was received from the local research ethics committee.

## Findings

Three main themes emerged from the qualitative data. They were

'Pain: processing or passing on?'
'A system of social defences.'
'What helps?'

The findings reported in this paper refer to one of the themes only (i.e. 'pain: processing or passing on). Only where there is overlap between themes, will any reference be made to systems of social defences or interventions that help with managing the nurse–patient relationship with people diagnosed with PDs. Full accounts of themes of 'a system of social defences' and 'what helps' will be published at a later date.

### *Pain: processing or passing on?*

The theme of 'pain: processing or passing on?' is presented in this paper. This theme reflects the basic emotional brutality of experience within the nurse–patient relationship, whereby the raw and penetrating emotional pain of abuse appears to suffuse interpersonal transactions. The nature of therapeutic response employed by nurses appeared to be determined by their prior clinical training which in turn was informed by the apparent model of care operating within the services they worked in.

### *The onslaught*

Nurses described occasions when they felt battered by an onslaught of emotional abuse and pain. Nurses described 'incident after incident' of violence, self-harm and verbal abuse (including sexualised and racial abuse) occurring in rapid succession in the forensic services. This typically occurred when a number of patients engaged in painful transacting, either simultaneously or one after another, leaving the nurse overwhelmed:

> In fact it was very, very disturbing for me that evening, very, very disturbing and I felt that I needed some time out because I could feel it within me. In as much as we are trained to contain all this I think it gets to a point where there is only so much that you can take. If it keeps coming and coming and coming and coming you just need time to be off the ward to reflect on why this presentation is going on and try and make some sense out of it. (RN, WEMSS)

### *Words hurt*

Experiences of pain or abuse were often verbally inflicted through threats, denigrating remarks and worst of all, personalised attacks:

> ... that was the first time that I actually broke down and cried after a patient had attacked me like that. There was a sense of aggression as well, physical aggression. She was banging and kicking the office door but I don't think the physical really bothered me, I think the personal things you know, that she said, because of what was said about my coming here and who had been moved out. I think it was quite personal to me and I find it quite difficult to work with .... (RN, WEMSS)

Nurses described feeling threatened and belittled at these times, with patients often swearing at them using the strongest forms of profanity. Episodes of verbal abuse usually took place in full view of others, which resulted in the nurse feeling exposed, vulnerable, humiliated and angry. Hate-fuelled words by patients could feel penetrative, and were reported from the perspective of obtruding through nurses' metaphoric protective barriers:

> You develop armour to protect yourself from those words but sometimes they just come straight through. (RN, WEMSS)

During interviews, the lasting emotional impact and distress of verbal attacks on a nurse could be evident by the way they described an incident. For example, the following quote was from a nurse who described an experience that occurred while being required to remain positioned outside of a room maintaining constant engagement and observation with a patient who was secluded following a risk incident. The lasting and apparently unprocessed impact was evident by the nature of their recall, which was mostly spoken as if by the patient:

> You bloody bitch, you wanker, you fat piece of shit!" You know, I was taking all that abuse. Sometimes, I find it really challenging, like with that patient, he really abused me you know. "I'm going to tell the doctors, I'm going to tell everyone that you come into my room and that you, you, you, like to suck my cock, you like to suck my dick, you, you, you bastard, you, you, you bitch I'm coming after you when I'm released by the Mental Health Review Tribunal. I'm going to kill you. I've got contacts outside of the hospital. I will make sure I know what type of car you are driving and I'm going to make sure you disappear." You are receiving all of this and on top of that, spitting at you. And then after that he makes a complaint against me when he's out of seclusion, to the Mental Health Act Commissioners that I was abusive to him when he was in the seclusion room. (RN DSPD)

### *Accusations and complaints*

Emotional brutality also occurred through interactions that were not so immediately violent, such as by making formal accusations or complaints about nurses who felt the process to be used for grievances other than those stated in the formal complaint. This was a phenomenon associated with the DSPD unit, perhaps mirroring the patients' histories of extensive contact with the criminal justice system including uncomfortable exposure and scrutiny involved in being 'brought down', by the process of accusation, arrest, investigation, charges and conviction:

> Yes, I mean with this complaint going through at the moment I'm feeling low. I'm probably feeling the lowest I've ever felt. (RN DSPD)

### *Self-harm*

Self-harm by patients elicited strong, painful feelings in nurses. For example, they described feeling 'worthless', 'useless' or 'a failure' when a patient self-harmed. The emotional impact on primary nurses was typically severe and negative:

> One always stays with me because I almost went off work with the stress of working with her and even thinking about it you know. I can still feel those same feelings I mean her self-harm was chronically severe, she used to burn herself all over her body and I was her primary nurse and it was intolerable. What she did to herself was horrible, it was horrible. (RN, TC)

Nurses working in forensic services described being required to maintain continuous engagement and observations with patients who were assessed to be acting dangerously to the point of presenting a severe risk to themselves. In these situations, self-harm was often intertwined with behaviours that presented a risk to other people. Nurses were therefore required to ensure that they were able to see the patient and what they were doing at all times. This could require bearing witness to horrific acts. The emotional impact was such that nurses described barely managing to remain in their professional roles:

> She grabbed a CD, split it in two, dug it well deep into her skin and in fact at that point if it had happened to me outside, maybe I would have just walked away because I couldn't bear seeing the blood gushing out … I couldn't bear watching it. (RN, WEMSS)

Of all the painful, challenging behaviours described in this study, self-harm was most strongly identified by patients and nurses as being part of an individual's repertoire of complex care seeing strategies:

> Every night, every night I worked she would present me at whatever hour of the morning with a self-harm. It could sometimes be steri-stripped but sometimes it would mean she had to go up to the ER to have it stitched erm and therefore she got the time with me although it was destructive because of my angry feelings, she got the time with me. (RN, TC)

> I find that incredibly difficult because at times I've actually thought in my head: "Well if they're harming every day and it seems to be OK and they're the ones getting the attention why don't I just go back to it?" "Why don't I just go back to cutting myself? Why don't I just go back to starving myself all day, all night, all year whatever because then maybe people will see that I'm struggling." But they don't seem to see that you're struggling if you don't act destructively. (Patient, TC)

### *Violence to others*

In keeping with the pattern of launching into multiple forms of painful relating that drew nurses in, violent behaviour was frequently accompanied by verbal abuse, accusations, rejection and personalised attacks. In this study, physical assaults on nurses were associated only with the WEMSS:

> It's just happened to me. My patient was, she, she's been calling me all sorts of names; "Fuck this and you piss off!" All sorts of stuff and eventually tried to attack another patient and you try dividing them and you're the one who gets kicked and then she starts the rejection process … "You can fuck off because you don't care for me. You care for them. You just go out and be in love with the rest of them! You don't like me …". (RN, WEMSS)

### *How nurses work with the onslaught*

From nurses' descriptions of how they worked with the onslaught of emotional or physical pain, a distinct approach emerged from those who worked in the TC and the WEMSS. This approach was often described by the nurses in terms of 'containing' the patients' emotional distress. All nurses who described working in this way reported that they had received some post-qualifying training in psychodynamic nursing theory and practice. Importantly, they described working in services for which psychoanalytic or psychodynamic approaches were integral to the model of care.

### *Containing*

The containing approach drew on psychoanalytic theories and practices such as Bion's (1962) theory of psychological containment. As such, the nurses understood their first task to be to interpret the negative emotional impact they experienced from the perspective of the patients' own painful feelings that were so overwhelming that they could not process them through thought or articulate them verbally. The patient was therefore understood to be unconsciously projecting these feelings onto the nurse, using risk behaviours to add extra purchase:

> I think sometimes these projections are something that the patient owns but is not able to process and make sense of it but pushes it into me to try to process for her. (RN, WEMSS)

The crucial component of containment that nurses performed via the use of self was to process through thought and conscious awareness what the patient was unable to do themselves. Doing so successfully could serve as a guide for the nurse in terms of both indicating what the patient is struggling with and how to respond therapeutically. Therefore, in the case of the containing nurses, the emotional pain experienced during interactions with patients was used to inform their approach to and delivery of nursing care:

> They could be hurting, you know and they want you to hurt as well, as much as they are hurting you know. It's a way of telling you: "This is the way that I am hurting." You need to stop and think: "Oh no, this is what she is trying to say to me, she's got problems. I need to get in there and try to work with her through whatever is going on". (RN, WEMSS)

While recognising the importance of understanding projective processes and communications, some nurses were able to recognise that the interaction with patients also included aspects of themselves which may be contributing, stressing the relevance of self-awareness:

> I think it's a mistake to blame work for everything you feel. It's also a mistake when a patient is telling you you're no good, assuming that is automatically a projection from a patient. Sometimes we are no good, you know. Sometimes being objective tells us that we do do things wrong so you do have to question yourself rather than ascribing everything automatically to projection. (RN, TC)

Nurses who employed a containing approach described how walking away, avoiding or otherwise not engaging with the onslaught of emotional pain would be the easier option and that mobilising internal capacity to effect containment did require substantial conscious effort and emotional resource on their part:

> I think rather than see personality disorders as a waste of time or self-harm as manipulative it's a communication of some sort and you have to try and understand what that communication is even if you don't really want to, even if you dread coming in to work with this particular patient. (RN, TC)

### *Attachment and care seeking*

Containing nurses recognised that they were sometimes 'on the receiving end' of an onslaught but regarded this as central to the nurse–patient relationship with people diagnosed with PDs. Indeed, the onslaught was often regarded as having an attachment function and perceived by nurses as a particularly complex method of care seeking. They also understood that what informed the patients' difficulties with care seeking was the combination of an internal drive to seek help when struggling, which was inextricably linked to their lack of faith in nurses to provide them with the help they needed. This was associated with early attachment experiences that had now left them, during periods of emotional dysregulation for example, believing that care would not be forthcoming either because they were not perceived as worthy by those who could provide it or that those who could provide care would not elect to do so or are incapable of doing so (Bowlby, 1973):

> They'll push you. "I don't want you. I want to stay in my bedroom in peace. I don't want you." They'll shut the door. They'll bang it right in front of you but they actually need you at that point. I have seen some of the patients coming back to you and saying to you: "Look, when I'm very distressed I tell you I don't want you but actually I do need you". (RN, WEMSS)

Patients also described the difficulties experienced both with their feelings, and with eliciting care from nurses to help them prior to engaging in destructive behaviours. For example, the quote below is from a patient describing her state of mind prior to self-harming:

> I'll go to my room and I'll be thinking over it and I'll be trying to think what can I say to the staff and my problems seem so complex that I think the staff just wouldn't understand. It seems so complicated from where it started and what happened and I feel like this or I feel let down or whatever and it's just too much of a jumbled up mess to sort out and I don't think the staff can possibly understand. (Patient, WEMSS)

Most strikingly, patients described the painful impact on them of unexpected separations and abrupt endings in their therapeutic relationships or indeed, therapeutic interactions with nurses as the following quotes from patients reflect:

> And I find that really, really difficult and it's the same with my original primary nurse who was only there for six weeks while I was here when she left. Oh, I felt like I was hit in the face with a sledge hammer. It was really, really difficult .... (Patient TC)

> And I have to agree as well like when you're talking and they're called off or you know, or you want some continuity regarding the nursing staff on your ward and they come in and you think: "Oh, it's good to see you, we can have a chat" and then

> they're redirected somewhere else and then some stranger ends up on the ward and you think 'Well, what's all that about?' So, I find all that difficult, I find all that hard to deal with and I don't think that's just my personal opinion, I've heard like many, many patients on many of the wards on here who don't like all this re-directing staff. If the staff come in to work on this ward, this is where they should work. Not directing them all over, looking for staff, do you know what I mean? That's my personal opinion. (Patient, DSPD)

Both patients and nurses in their different ways consistently indicated that an approach to the nurse–patient relationship that recognised and responded to the PD patients' sensitivity to attachment related experiences, was clinically relevant and personally valuable in terms of supporting the patients' recovery. Included, was recognition of the ever present pressure to re-enact traumatic attachment experiences:

> ... it does make you question your ability to actually work in this environment and you can easily get into huge trouble because if you're not able to understand what you're doing and process your own feelings you might end up being a big abuser, if you like. You know, acting as an abuser, if you're not processing your feelings properly. So, if she rejects you, you might end up rejecting her back and then you become not a carer; you become an abuser. So, I do try as much as possible to try and process my own feelings and thoughts and behaviours but there's times when I do struggle. (RN, WEMSS)

Pressure on nurses to re-enact traumatic attachment experiences may be as perpetrator, which is described in the above quote. However, it may also be as victim. Nurses described examples of patients apparently attempting to pull them out of their professional role by interpersonal strategies of domination and control:

> We have a patient who likes to shout at you, order you around and so forth .... (RN, DSPD)

When patients' interpersonal style inclined towards pressurising nurses to assume a victim role, this was contained by nurses adopting what they often described as a 'challenging' stance:

> ... You have to see through that and say "Look, hold up, you shouldn't speak to me like that. I'm not going to let you speak to me like that. It's not appropriate. You know its not appropriate .... (RN, DSPD)

In order to avoid re-enacting abusive dynamics as either victim or perpetrator but instead provide psychological containment and a secure, therapeutic relationship for patients, the nurses reported requiring significant support. In particular, they required support to manage boundaries within the therapeutic relationship given the pressure to lose their professional footing and adopt anti-therapeutic roles, which would in all likelihood result in their participating in a re-enactment of a patient's prior trauma or index offence, or both. Support that nurses described as being essential for establishing and maintaining sufficient resilience to effectively undertake the incredible emotional labour inherent in managing the nurse–patient relationship with this complex population included training and a secure emotional base from where they sought their own form of care in the form of somewhere to think and someone to think with. This could be achieved by the availability of 'containing spaces' such as the reflective practice and supervision sessions, which were an integral part of all the services included in this study:

> I think if you are to rely on your own resources you are likely to burn out in this environment ... you live with these patients. They come in here for a very long period of time. You live with them so to receive attacks from them on repetitive occasions, not having an identified outlet makes it very difficult so one of the things that I find useful is being in a group or even 1:1 supervision and venting out my feelings and then getting support in processing some of those feelings. (RN, WEMSS)

## Discussion

The findings from this study confirm those from other studies in that nurses' experiences of managing the nurse–patient relationship with people diagnosed with PDs are often pain-ridden and for that reason, constitute tremendous emotional labour (Bowers, 2002; Woollaston & Hixenbaugh, 2008). Additionally, by combining the patients' perspective with that of nurses working in specialist PD services, this study further clarifies the interpersonal processes involved; identifying, in particular that behind the destructive, alienating presentations of PD patients, exists a plea for understanding, care and support from nurses (Cremin et al., 1995; McMillan & Aiyegbusi, 2009).

It is hypothesised that some sources of enduring emotional pain emanate from patients' early biographies and may best be understood in terms of unprocessed traumatic sequelae of their early experiences with caregivers. Highly sensitive to attachment phenomena, emotional dysregulation is triggered by intense attachment experiences and appears to evoke anxieties that emerge within the nurse–patient relationship: often characterised by perceptions of rejection or abandonment. Early experiences may also have left some people compromised and vulnerable in terms of being unable to clearly express their emotional needs for the purpose of seeking care. Fearful of the neglect or rejection they expect to receive based on past attachment experiences, and being unable to articulate their needs or regulate their emotions, they generate an onslaught of emotional pain. This is given extra purchase through a repertoire of destructive behaviours. One attachment-oriented dimension of this appears to be an unconscious attempt to communicate the need for care by projecting forms of distress onto, and sometimes into, nursing staff themselves. The unconscious purpose being to communicate the pain they are feeling through perhaps the only medium felt to be available. That is through emotional impact (Casement, 1985).

Another attachment oriented dimension of the patients' onslaught of painful interpersonal behaviours appears to be that of increasing proximity and securing interpersonal contact with nurses through various methods of pain generation. Working therapeutically with this onslaught is extremely challenging but nevertheless seems core to the nursing role in such circumstances. Depending on their clinical and emotional capacity in conjunction with the nature of support and training available, nurses may either process the distress or pass it back to the patient with the latter style contributing to an ever escalating, destructive cycle.

In keeping with the views previously expressed by people diagnosed with PD (Castillo, 2003; NIMHE, 2003), their sensitivity, dysregulated emotions and accompanying destructive or risk behaviours may be understood in terms of an activated attachment system and consequent attachment behaviours in those who are compromised by negative developmental histories, and by residing or being detained in an institutional setting that they experience to be unresponsive. However, as has been suggested in this study, informing the nurse–patient relationship via theories of attachment and psychological containment may provide a hopeful way forward, which will serve to support recovery with this challenging, vulnerable and often excluded population. Doing so, however, requires significant investment in psychodynamic training and supervision for nurses if they are to understand their work in terms of skilled interpersonal process rather than to perceive themselves as legitimised emotional punch bags to be repeatedly assaulted with no purpose or end in sight. Recognising the absence of training for clinicians to work therapeutically with people diagnosed with PDs, the Department of Health and Ministry of Justice jointly commissioned the development of a national training and development framework in 2008, which is named the Knowledge and Understanding Framework. This co-produced and delivered training includes an understanding of PDs from a trauma and attachment theory perspective, provides support to understand the management of boundaries and the provision of psychological containment, emphasising the role of reflective practice and supervision to build resilience in individual practitioners and teams (Institute of Mental Health, University of Nottingham, 2009). This training which can be accessed as part of a pathway from basic awareness to B.Sc. and M.Sc., would appear to offer an effective response to the development requirements described by the participants in this study.

## Acknowledgements

Acknowledgements are made to all those who agreed to take part in this study, and to the managers of the research settings who allowed access. Grateful thanks to Vicky Franks, Janet Holmshaw and FeryGazy for their encouragement, advice and assistance at different stages of the research and to Gillian Kelly who co-facilitated the focus groups.

## Disclosure statement

No potential conflict of interest was reported by the author.

## References

Adshead, G. (1998). Psychiatric staff as attachment figures. Understanding management problems in psychiatric services in the light of attachment theory. *British Journal of Psychiatry*, *172*, 64–69. doi:10.1192/bjp.172.1.64

American Psychiatric Association. (2013). *Diagnostic and statistical manual of mental disorders* (5th ed.). Washington, DC: Author.

Bion, W. R. (1962). A theory of thinking. *International Journal of Psycho-Analysis, 43*, 4–5.

Bland, A. R., Tudor, G., & Mcneil Whitehouse, D. M. (2007). Nursing care of inpatients with borderline personality disorder. *Perspectives in Psychiatric Care, 43*, 204–212. doi:10.1111/j.1744-6163.2007.00135.x

Bowers, L. (2002). *Dangerous and severe personality disorder: Response and role of the psychiatric team*. London: Routledge.

Bowlby, J. (1973). *Attachment and loss volume 2: Separation, anger and anxiety*. London: The Tavistock Institute of Human Relations.

Bray, J. (1999). An ethnographic study of psychiatric nursing. *Journal of Psychiatric and Mental Health Nursing, 6*, 297–305. doi:10.1046/j.1365-2850.1999.00215.x

Casement, P. (1985). *On learning from the patient*. Oxford: Routledge.

Castillo, H. (2003). *Personality disorder: Temperament or trauma?* London: Jessica Kingsley.

Cremin, D., Lemmer, B., & Davison, S. (1995). The efficacy of a nursing challenge to patients: Testing a new intervention to decrease self-harm behaviour in severe personality disorder. *Journal of Psychiatric and Mental Health Nursing, 2*, 237–246. doi:10.1111/j.1365-2850.1995.tb00063.x

Department of Health. (1999). *Report of the committee of inquiry into the personality disorder unit, Ashworth Special Hospital*. London: The Stationary Office.

Department of Health. (2002). *Into the mainstream: Consultation paper about women's mental health strategy*. London: Author.

Department of Health. (2003). *Mainstreaming gender. Implementing the women's mental health strategy*. London: Author.

Department of Health, Home Office, Her Majesty's Prison Service. (2004). *Dangerous and severe personality disorder (DSPD) high security services planning and delivery guide*. London: Home Office.

Department of Health and National Offender Management Service. (2011). *Response to the offender personality disorder consultation*. Leeds: DH/NOMS.

Evans, M., & Franks, V. (1997). Psychodynamics as an aid to clear thinking about patients. *Nursing Times, 93*, 50–53.

Fallon, P. (2003). Travelling through the system: The lived experience of people with borderline personality disorder in contact with psychiatric services. *Journal of Psychiatric and Mental Health Nursing, 10*, 393–401. doi:10.1046/j.1365-2850.2003.00617.x

Fonagy, P., & Bateman, A. W. (2007). Mentalizing and borderline personality disorder. *Journal of Mental Health, 16*, 83–101. doi:10.1080/09638230601182045

Fraser, K., & Gallop, R. (1993). Nurses' confirming/disconfirming responses to patients diagnosed with borderline personality disorder. *Archives of Psychiatric Nursing, 7*, 336–341. doi:10.1016/0883-9417(93)90051-W

Gallop, R., & O'Brien, L. (2003). Re-establishing psychodynamic theory as foundational knowledge for psychiatric/mental health nursing. *Issues in Mental Health Nursing, 24*, 213–227. doi:10.1080/01612840305302

Goodman, C. M. (1987). The Delphi technique: A critique. *Journal of Advanced Nursing, 12*, 729–734.

Hare, R. D. (1991). *The psychopathy checklist – Revised*. Toronto: Multi Health Systems.

Hare, R. D. (2003). *Manual for the revised psychopathy checklist*. Toronto: Multi Health Systems.

Herman, J. L. (1992). *Trauma and recovery: From domestic violence to political terror*. London: Basic Books.

Herman, J. L., & van der Kolk, B. A. (1987). Traumatic antecedents of borderline personality disorder. In B. A. van der Kolk (Ed.), *Psychological trauma* (pp. 111–126). Washington, DC: American Psychiatric Press.

Husserl, E. (1900/1970). *Logical investigations – Volume 1*. Oxford: Routledge.

Institute of Mental Health, University of Nottingham. (2009). *Working effectively with personality disorder: The new KUF framework*. Nottingham: Institute of Mental Health.

James, P. D., & Cowman, S. (2007). Psychiatric nurses' knowledge, experience and attitudes towards clients with borderline personality disorder. *Journal of Psychiatric and Mental Health Nursing*, *14*, 670–678. doi:10.1111/j.1365-2850.2007.01157.x

Jones, A. C. (2005). Transference, counter-transference and repetition: Some implications for nursing practice. *Journal of Clinical Nursing*, *14*, 1177–1184. doi:10.1111/j.1365-2702.2005.01309.x

Linehan, M. (1993). *Cognitive behavioural treatment of borderline personality disorder*. New York, NY: Guilford.

Markham, D. (2003). Attitudes towards patients with a diagnosis of borderline personality disorder: Social rejection and dangerousness. *Journal of Mental Health*, *12*, 595–612. doi:10.1080/09638230310001627955

Markham, D., & Trower, P. (2003). The effects of the psychiatric label 'borderline personality disorder' on nursing staff's perceptions and causal attributions for challenging behaviours. *British Journal of Clinical Psychology*, *42*, 243–256. doi:10.1348/014466503607033666

Mason, T., Hall, R., Caulfied, M., & Melling, K. (2010). Forensic nurses' perceptions of labels of mental illness and personality disorder: Clinical versus management issues. *Journal of Psychiatric and Mental Health Nursing*, *17*, 131–140. doi:10.1111/j.1365-2850.2009.01483.x

McAndrew, S., & Warne, T. (2005). Cutting across boundaries: A case study using feminist praxis to understand the meanings of self-harm. *International Journal of Mental Health Nursing*, *14*, 172–180. doi:10.1111/j.1440-0979.2005.00378.x

McMillan, S., & Aiyegbusi, A. (2009). Crying out for care. In A. Aiyegbusi & J. Clarke–Moore (Eds.), *Therapeutic relationships with offenders: An introduction to the psychodynamics of forensic mental health nursing* (pp. 171–186). London: JKP.

Murphy, N., & McVey, D. (2003). The challenge of nursing personality-disordered patients. *The British Journal of Forensic Practice*, *5*, 3–19. doi:10.1108/14636646200300002

National Institute for Mental Health in England. (2003). *Personality disorder: No longer a diagnosis of exclusion. Policy implementation guidance for the development of services for people with personality disorder*. London: Department of Health.

O'Kelly, G. (1998). Countertransference in the nurse–patient relationship: A review of the literature. *Journal of Advanced Nursing*, *28*, 391–397. doi:10.1046/j.1365-2648.1998.00638.x

Peplau, H. E. (1952). *Interpersonal relations in nursing*. New York, NY: Putnams.

Ramon, S., Castillo, H., & Morant, N. (2001). Experiencing personality disorder: A participative research. *International Journal of Social Psychiatry*, *47*(4), 1–15. doi:10.1177/002076400104700401

Richman, J. (1998). Ceremonial order and moral reasoning in a ward for psychopaths. In T. Mason & D. Mercer (Eds.), *Critical perspectives in forensic care: Inside out* (pp. 146–170). London: Macmillan Press.

Ritchie, J., & Spencer, L. (1994). Qualitative data analysis for applied policy research. In A. Bryman & R. G. Burgess (Eds.), *Analysing qualitative data* (pp. 173–194). London: Routledge.

Ritchie, J., Spencer, L., & O'Connor, W. (2003). Carrying out qualitative analysis. In J. Ritchie & J. Lewis (Eds.), *Qualitative research practice: A guide for social science students and researchers* (pp. 219–262). London: Sage.

Rogers, B., & Dunne, E. (2011). 'They told me I had this personality disorder ... all of a sudden I was wasting their time': Personality disorder and the inpatient experience. *Journal of Mental Health, 20*, 226–233. doi:10.3109/09638237.2011.556165

Silverman, D. (2000). *Doing qualitative research: A practical handbook*. London: Sage.

Stockwell, F. (1972). *The unpopular patient*. Royal College of Nursing Research Project. Series 1. No 2. London: RCN.

Warne, T., & McAndrew, S. (2007). Bordering on insanity: Misnomer, reviewing the case of condemned women. *Journal of Psychiatric and Mental Health Nursing, 14*, 155–162. doi:10.1111/j.1365-2850.2007.01058.x

Winship, G. (1998). Intensive care psychiatric nursing – Psychoanalytic perspectives 1. *Journal of Psychiatric and Mental Health Nursing, 5*, 361–365. doi:10.1046/j.1365-2850.1998.00150.x

Woollaston, K., & Hixenbaugh, P. (2008). 'Destructive whirlwind': Nurses perceptions of patients diagnosed with borderline personality disorder. *Journal of Psychiatric and Mental Health Nursing, 15*, 703–709. doi:10.1111/j.1365-2850.2008.01275.x

# Safety in numbers: group therapy-based index offence work in secure psychiatric care

Gwen Adshead

*Department of Forensic Psychiatry, Fareham ,UK*

In this paper, I discuss the provision of dynamically based index offence group work for forensic patients who are detained in long-stay residential secure care. I discuss the benefits of reflective, attachment theory-based therapies as complementary to the other models of therapy that are offered to forensic patients. In particular, I discuss the relevance of this type of psychotherapy to *index offence work*, using the example of a reflective recovery-based therapy group for forensic patients who have killed. I discuss the relevance of identity and agency change in the narratives of group members, illustrating with quotes from the group. I conclude with comment about resistance to such work, and the impact on therapists of working with the trauma of homicide perpetration.

## Introduction

In liberal societies, offenders are offered rehabilitation during their period of detention. In the USA, Canada and most European countries, this has led to the development of therapeutic and psycho-educational programmes for offenders, both in prisons and in the community. Group therapies have been offered to offenders in prison since the 1950s (e.g. Landers, Macphail, & Simpson, 1954; Mackwood, 1951; McCorkle, 1949, 1953); and in 1964, Michael Foulkes first suggested that group analysis might be beneficial for people he called socially 'deviant'. Group work is still the main form of psychological therapeutic intervention available to prisoners, and group-based cognitive therapy is recommended for antisocial men and women by the National Institute for Clinical Excellence (2009).

In this paper, I discuss the use of psychodynamic group therapy as an important treatment modality for offenders with mental illnesses, who are detained in secure psychiatric services. I argue that this is an intervention which should be available to all offender patients who can use it. I base my claim on my experience of offering such therapy as part of a programme of group therapies that offer a range of therapy groups in a variety of modalities. There has been comparatively little discussion on the use of psychodynamic group therapy in forensic psychiatric services; papers by Cox (1976) and Welldon (1993) are honourable exceptions and my work has been greatly influenced by theirs.

The comparative lack of discussion may be related to a confusion between technique and process. There are important theoretical differences between delivering a psychological technique in a group format [as is common for dialectical behaviour therapy (DBT) and cognitive behaviour therapy (CBT)] and using the relational processes of being together in a group to facilitate psychological change; space does not allow me to discuss these differences here. I have no doubt that the different psychological techniques are complementary, and all forensic patients need to be offered therapies in groups, if only because of the essentially pro-social nature of group therapy, and I discuss this further below.

However, I want to argue specifically that psychodynamic therapy that offers space for reflection on conscious and less-conscious processes is essential for offenders who have damaged their social identities by their offences, and who need to demonstrate to themselves and others that they have thought about their offending and its consequences. Forensic psychiatric patients are expected to spend time thinking about the offence that led to their detention, what is called (in the jargon of prisons) the 'index offence'. As people with mental illness, they are also invited to participate in their own recovery. I want to describe here how psychodynamic group work can act as a vehicle for both 'index offence work' and recovery. I will discuss how psychodynamic reflective groups support the recovery paradigm through an emphasis on user-led narrative, and how groups support risk reduction by helping people explore their experience of choosing to act in the way they did, and their sense of responsibility for their offending.

By reflective psychodynamic group psychotherapy, I mean those group therapeutic techniques that emphasise the development of the capacity to reflect on one's own mind and the minds of others, and use group processes to do so. In this sense, they are groups that attempt to enhance participants' capacity to *mentalise* (Allen & Fonagy, 2006; Fonagy & Adshead, 2012). Groups that emphasise mentalising differ from traditional group analytic therapy in terms of more direct activity by therapists in the process of the group, and an explicit focus on the theme of mentalising (Karterud & Bateman, 2012). However, mentalising groups are similar to traditional group techniques in that therapists allow the dialogue in the group to be led primarily by the patients, not the therapists, and there is no agenda to the group process. This does not mean the groups are 'unstructured' (a common misperception); in fact, they are highly structured in terms of time, boundaries and focus. However, they do not have pre-set topics for discussion, as is common in manualised groups.

What psychodynamic groups can also do is offer group members a chance to generate and reflect on the narratives of their lives and identities, i.e. the way that people tell the stories of their lives and their choices. To illustrate this claim, I use material from a long-running psychodynamic reflective therapy group for men who have killed when mentally ill. The group participants are patients in a secure psychiatric hospital who have been offered therapy as part of a groupwork programme. When patients join the groups, they give permission for their material to be used in anonymous and unidentifiable ways, and I wish to express my gratitude to them here. Pseudonyms are used throughout. I am also grateful to my colleagues in the groupwork services who made the development of these groups possible.

## Background: groups as pro-social processes

Human beings are evolved from primates who live in groups, and have identities based on belonging to groups. Group membership fosters parent–offspring attachment, and also peer–peer and sexual relationships within the group. Group membership protects its members and confers good health and extended life; for both humans and non-human primates, social exclusion and isolation are associated with poor physical health and early death as well as violence towards others who are within the group membership (Steptoe, Shankar, Demakakos, & Wardle, 2013).

Neocortical brain volume is directly related to group size and the development of language in humans (Aiello & Dunbar, 1993). Our neocortical volume makes possible the development of a social mind: a mind that can conceive of others and allow relationships to form which support the existence of the group. Living in groups keeps us safe from external predators, and so the capacities of our social mind include the capacity to identify outsiders, as well as potential mates, competitors and allies within the group.

As Dunbar points out, the key function of the enhanced size of the neocortex is the development of language, because this allows for relationships to exist in mind and over time. Rather than relationships based on physical grooming, relationships can be based on signs and symbols that can be held in memory and carried across from place to place, so that physical contact is no longer necessary. This makes group membership reliant on both a mentalising capacity: keeping mind in mind and the capacity to 'speaking our language' as a means of connection.

It is no accident that those who get excluded from groups are those who cannot be empathic and mentalise; and those who cannot 'speak their minds', i.e. they lack the symbolic language and the words to describe their mental states and those of others. To be without language is to be anti-human; one thinks here of those feral children who never learn to be human. But by definition, those who cannot belong to human groups may be judged by others to be anti-human.

There are other ways of being excluded from human groups, and one way is to break the rules of the group. How human groups develop and maintain rules is a huge subject in its own right, and of course abuts onto other huge intellectual domains such as sociology, political science, philosophy and law. However, the key issue here is that for humans (as for other primates), breaking social rules leads to social exclusion. When a person breaks the rules, they are doing something to their social identity as well as expressing something important for themselves. When the rule-breaking involves violence to others (i.e. physical harm and the wish to hurt), then such violence causes a breach in the matrix and psychological 'walls' of the larger social group. The offender both drops out through the breach and is pushed out of the group. It is for this reason that the criminal law states that a criminal offence is an offence against the whole body politic, why crimes are defined by statute, and individual victims are not given primacy in criminal courts. The offence is against the large group as a whole, not just the individual victim. When one is hurt, all are hurt.

Pain and fear generate rage and hate. This is not just the gospel according to Yoda; it is good neurophysiological and neuropsychological science. A group member who frightens and threatens others will be excluded from his original group with enthusiasm that conveys fear and disgust, and mirrors the offender's own similar feelings. No doubt other mental mechanisms operate such as projection and envy, which assist the exclusion process. Although all of us may have lapses of mentalising and emotional processing, such that we experience thoughts or feelings of cruelty and destructiveness, nevertheless, the truth is that most people do not act on those thoughts and feelings, whether conscious or unconscious. Those who do have *crossed the line*: a reference to an invisible boundary that marks out group membership and identity. Having crossed the line, these men and women may never be able to go back to their original groups, and find themselves isolated and without a social context to which to attach.

In primate societies, animals who are not members of the group are either predator or prey; and this is precisely the situation that forensic patients find themselves in after they have committed offences. They are seen as both a threat to the large group or community to which they used to belong, and someone who is outside the human group, and is therefore a legitimate target. There is extensive evidence that forensic patients have histories of victimisation both before and after their offending histories began, and they are at risk of increased morbidity and early death.

My view is that group work programmes are vital in forensic services for reasons that relate both to patient welfare and risk reduction. First, therapy groups (of any sort) allow offenders to rejoin a group and be part of a pro-social process once more. This is not always an easy or comfortable process: a man in Broadmoor once said to me, *I don't want to be in a group with people like me.* But secure services are communities of the excluded: the unloved and the unlovable. To enable people to become more pro-social, they need to be able to belong to a group.

Second, forensic patients need to have space to explore the issue of exclusion and their experiences of being antisocial, or even anti-human. In therapeutic groups, men and women offenders can safely explore their antisocial selves;

accept their reality and then use the group as a pro-social space to transform. This is where the range of techniques is valuable: CBT and DBT allow patients to develop awareness of their own thoughts and thinking styles, and the possibility of change. Purely cognitively based groups (such as the Violent Offenders Programme) are valuable for the purely cognitive aspects of offending; for example, the antisocial beliefs that support offending. The Violent Offenders Programme challenges thinking processes such as 'It is right to get revenge' or 'Anger is uncontrollable.' However, such groups do not explore the group process itself as an aid to mentalising, and because the programmes were devised for prisoners (who are assumed to be in good mental health), they may be less appropriate for offenders with mental illnesses whose cognitions are disturbed by psychosis or severe mood disorder.

Furthermore, the Violent Offenders Programme can explore the general cognitions that promote violence, but cannot deal with specific personal and relational aspects of violence, such as the homicide of a loved one. They also do not address the lived experience of being an offender; what it is like to live with the new and unwelcome identity that follows conviction for fatal violence. Forensic patients also need therapeutic spaces where they can reflect deeply on their identity as offenders, in ways that help them manage high-risk affects such as shame and anger. My experience has been that men who have offended against someone they know need a reflective group that can offer a relational perspective to complement the individual cognitive perspective of the Violent Offenders Programme.

## How do reflective groups effect change: (i) coherence of self-narrative

A key aspect of psychological change after therapy is reflected in how people talk about themselves. A study of effective psychological therapy by Adler, Skalina, and McAdams (2008) found that people who experienced therapy as helpful demonstrated enhanced narrative coherence and a sense of agency. van Staden and Fulford (2004) describe increased use of the personal pronoun during the course of therapy, again suggesting an enhanced sense of agency.

A key concept is that of 'narrative coherence', which is described by many theorists. Work on attachment narratives has drawn on the work of Grice to define narrative coherence, and develop a linguistic analysis coding system for attachment narratives generated by an interview that explores the adult attachment system (George, Kaplan, & Main, 1985; Hesse, 2008). This literature has demonstrated that security of mind is revealed in the language used by the person speaking about their attachment experiences, and that there are distinct linguistic patterns associated with different forms of attachment insecurity. Detailed analysis of all aspects of language may help to identify psychopathological processes that are not conscious to the speaker. They adduce strongest evidence in relation to the effects of unresolved trauma and loss on language, e.g. long pauses or gaps in speech, odd associations or metaphors and lapses in monitoring of discourse. This work is complemented by other studies that have noted that changes of verb tense can be an indicator of high emotion or distress; for example, speaking in the present tense indicates that the speaker is experiencing their feelings in the present and distortion of temporal reality testing (Hashemi et al. 2008; Pillemer, Desroches, & Ebanks, 1997).

Highly disorganised and unresolved states of mind are associated with more severe clinical conditions, especially psychotic disorders (Schwannauer, 2013). What follows are random quotes from members of a group for men who have killed someone close to them. I have italicised those that I think have particular indicators of narrative incoherence, especially a sense of preoccupation with the offence, repetition of key phrases and the suggestion (not corrected by the speaker) that the victim is not actually dead.

> *I didn't kill anyone ... you can dig him up and ask him if you don't believe me ....*
>
> Being born and taking a life are similar. You will always remember
>
> When people ask me if I regret killing Mary I often say no. When I said yes, people were pleased.
>
> It's a private club for people who have killed a loved one. A life changing experience
>
> What I did was out of proportion
>
> *Can't remember the index, only bits of it. I was out of it ... a bit protective I suppose. I remember stabbing my [victim] in the head ... the noise of it, and then getting help. The ambulance coming ... I need my family to fill in the gaps*
>
> P1: Did you see on the news about the man who killed his wife while he was asleep?
> P2: He'll be devastated when he wakes up.
>
> *My mum was part of my index offence. I nearly murdered her, then I killed my dad and I nearly killed my mum.*
>
> My family are proud of what I have done. It was time for a change.
>
> *I killed my mum, my old dear*
>
> It was like the world falling away
>
> [In a discussion of visits] *I killed my mother so obviously I don't see her.*
>
> We talked for the first hour about my index offence. Thought I would feel like a school boy again but I didn't. I answered her questions as best I could. She doesn't know and sometimes maybe I don't know myself
>
> *It's psychological power. People you're close to can hurt you in ways your enemies only dream about.*
>
> *If I hadn't killed my girlfriend I would have been dead.*
>
> *I'm justified. My hands are clean. I did what I had to do. I can tell my dad I love him now. Our relationship is better since my offence.*
>
> [A discussion of a victim]

P1: *Do you think she was aware of what was going on? Did she know it was you?*
P2: *Yes, she knows.*

P1: *I was in a hole and had to dig myself out.*
P2: *How did you dig yourself out?*
P1: *Committing my offence I suppose.*

I note how many of these speakers drift into the present tense, and speak of their victims as if they were still alive. There is potential incoherence in the idea that life is better now after the offence; a key theme that deserves extensive reflection and consideration in relation to risk. If it is true that the homicide has led to some sustained psychological change for the better, then this would have significant bearing on risk. However, given the traumatic nature of homicide commission, therapists might be wary of such claims, and think they reflect unresolved distress and denial. Only repeated and extended discussions with the speaker, and others who have had a similar experience, will allow the therapist to come to a reasonable assessment of the risk: there is certainly no risk assessment tool that is reliable in this context.

In contrast, here is a quote from Jack, a group member with a diagnosis of chronic psychosis, who often mutters unintelligibly to himself. One of the therapists gently comments that they cannot hear very well what Jack is saying, and Jack responds very clearly:

> I was thinking about the lady I killed and how I would like to say sorry . . . when I killed my mum I was mentally ill, but . . . there was no reason for me to kill the second lady.

Note that Jack makes a very clear distinction between two different states of mind in relation to a homicide, and the relationship with these states of mind and reasons for killing, i.e. to kill with no reason is to do something for which one feels regret. We had not been talking about feeling sorry or regretful or anything like it, but these thoughts were clearly on Jack's mind. It was a very clear statement from a man who had been a member of a previous group, but had not been offered individual work because he was seen as psychotic and unable to use it.

Listening to others tell their story reduces the sense of shame and social isolation brought about by the offence, and enhances people's abilities to tell their story. What we aim for in these groups is an enhanced coherence of narrative about the index offence, and evidence that the group members are able to generate and maintain a 'secure' and coherent narrative of what they have done. In an earlier paper (Adshead, 2011), I suggested that offender patients arrive in forensic service with a 'cover story', which is often highly incoherent, e.g. 'she made me do it', 'the demons told me to'. The work of therapy is to gently dismantle this 'cover story' and help group members reorganise their experiences into a more coherent and realistic narratives that includes reflection on their illness and their relationship with the victim. This is vitally important work for homicide perpetrators in particular because it is likely that they will repeatedly be required to tell the 'story' of their index offence to future professionals and colleagues: people who are total strangers and who may be frightened of them. Being able to provide a clear and coherent narrative of the index offence is likely to enhance their progress on rehabilitation and recovery pathways.

## How do reflective groups effect change: (ii) agency and redemption

Work by Dan McAdams, a sociologist, suggests that our personality is constructed in different levels, and that psychological change takes place at the narrative level (McAdams & Pals, 2006). He has studied what he calls 'redemptive narratives', i.e. accounts of life after traumatic experiences, in which people describe how they have tried (and sometimes are still trying) to make 'good' out of an experience of pain and suffering. What seems to be important here is agency and ownership of change, both in terms of taking action but also in being able to reflect on that change (Landman, 2001).

Presser's (2013) work with gang members in prison found that they used language that emphasised their heroic nature, and minimised their offender status. Such language is typical of 'neutralisation discourses' (Sykes & Matza, 1957) in which what is 'neutralised' in these is the experience of negative feelings that might cause pain or distress in the offender, such as shame, guilt, anxiety or self-reproach. Like other human beings, most offenders want to see themselves as 'good' people who have made mistakes, or been provoked into doing wrong. Psychological processes (both intrapersonal and interpersonal) that encourage the ownership of responsibility and agency for wrong-doing may be painful to experience, and generate negative affects of shame and grief that have to be endured and perhaps reluctantly accommodated into an offender's sense of identity.

Professionals working with offenders in rehabilitation programmes hope that offenders who can 'own' their agency and responsibility for offending are less likely to re-offend. Although this hope intuitively accords with cultural and religious norms, there is surprisingly little research to support it. One study by Maruna (2001) does provide some empirical evidence that ownership of personal responsibility for choices made is associated with desisting from crime. Maruna examined the narratives generated by two groups of offenders: those who had desisted from crime and those who had not. The 'desisters' generated narratives of themselves that emphasised their sense of a 'previous' offending self which was not their 'real' self; that there was an 'old me' and a 'new me' that were both connected and distinct. They also used language that indicated that they experienced a sense of agency and ownership in terms of making changes to their lives, e.g. 'It's down to me to change the way I act.' In contrast, the 'persisters' (who continued to offend) used language that suggested that they experienced themselves in a passive way, as people to whom things just 'happened'. They described a sense of waiting for something to change their lives, and implied that they were helpless to affect their futures.

Maruna's work echoes Adler's work cited above: that a failure to see oneself as agentic and influential in the world leads to a type of stuckness and passivity. This work echoes that of O'Connor (2000) who carried out a series of interviews with prisoners who had perpetrated serious violence. She found that these offenders (all male, and without mental illness problems) place themselves on what she called 'a continuum of agency'. In the homicide groups, the therapists are active in listening out for ownership of offending and agency in the index offence. Take, for example, the following quote from a group member:

> I feel I'm stuck in my previous age... the age I was when I did my offence... Time's passing here and there are things I'm not doing.. I want to capture time with magazines and pictures to record what I was doing when I was here... What will it be like in 10 years time? Where will we be? What will I think on my deathbed about this time?

Here is a speaker who is actively reflecting on time, and the possibilities of thinking differently in the future about himself and his offence. He can own agency for the 'offence' but cannot name it (i.e. 'when I did my offence', not 'when I killed...'). He wants to be 'doing' something and wants to be able to record and prove he was 'doing'. Although the language is quite fresh and coherent (as described above), this excerpt reads as if the speaker is emphasising 'doing' not 'being', which may suggest that he is still struggling with his identity as a homicide perpetrator. This hypothesis may be supported by the fact that the speaker did drop out of the group some time after this excerpt, but did return and re-engage after about a year. He was able to say that (*inter alia*) he had found being in the group with other people like him difficult because of the mirror effect of seeing other people who he did not always warm to.

In the group, we are trying to help the men move from the passive to the active voice, a process first described by Cox (1976). Cox notes how the recovery of the agency process is identifiable in the use of language:

> I don't know what you are talking about.
> It wasn't me.
> It was me, but I was mentally ill when I did it.
> I did it when I was mentally ill.
> I did it.

Cox (1976) refers to this as a 'scala integrata', but I think it may be better to see each group as a step along a Via Dolorosa, where every mental footstep is painful, and the therapist's job is to keep the patient company. In this sense, the recovery process for forensic patients can be very painful indeed, and we are always very aware of the risk of suicidal feelings emerging, given what is known about the extended risk of suicide in homicide perpetrators (Liettu et al., 2010).

Ferrito, Vetere, Adshead, and Moore (2012) carried out a qualitative analysis of narratives generated by men who have attended our homicide group. She explicitly used Dan McAdams' ideas about redemption in her analysis, and found that this theme recurred in many narratives. Repeatedly, men described a wish that they could do something good for others in the future; some action that would make some recompense for the damage they had done. One man in particular poignantly expressed a wish that he might make something of himself in the future so 'that two lives will not have been lost, and [the victim] will not have died in vain'.

I have commented elsewhere that these men are like survivors of a disaster where they were the disaster (Adshead, 2003). Trauma survivors are no longer encouraged to go over every last detail and expose themselves afresh to distress, in a painful exposure paradigm. Rather, there has been an acknowledgement that instead of going over the past, there is a need to reorganise the present in a way which integrates both the past and the future into a way of being 'now'. In this way, there can be some sort of transformation from one identity into another with the possibility of growth and development (Niemeyer, 2004). This is a process that Garland (1993) has called 'getting on with it, not getting over it'.

As described earlier, such transformation narratives have been called 'redemptive' (McAdams, Josselson, & Lieblich, 2001). We also explore the extent to which the killer identity can be given up, or transformed into something which is not completely defined by the past. However, the men and the therapists are all aware that this is not completely up to them to decide, and so it may not be possible for these men to leave that identity behind, even if the homicide is now a decade or more ago. Society (either in the form of the Justice administration or the media) will not let them forget, and some of them have continuing and complex relationships with the families that they altered irrevocably by their actions. We have seen that the social universe of these men is altered forever when they kill; and as another patient said to me:

> You can be an ex-bus driver but you can't be an ex-murderer.

A possible reason for the lack of published literature on group work with people who have killed (especially those who have killed someone close to them) is that the story to be written is essentially an incoherent one of contrasting identities. On the one hand, these people are homicide perpetrators, and this may be their own adopted defining identity (Hillbrand & Young, 2004). On the other hand, they are also victims of trauma, who have been suddenly and terribly bereaved. In a group context, they are people who are simultaneously fearsome perpetrators and traumatised victims. One of the tasks of the group is to integrate these two, often polarised, aspects of the group and its members, and to pose the question: how do you survive a disaster when you are the disaster?

## Issues for therapists: resistance and trauma

'Offender recovery' is defined by Drennan and Alred (2013) as 'coming to terms with having offended, perceiving the need to change one's attitudes and beliefs that gave rise to offending and which support the future risk of re-offending, and accepting the social and personal consequences of having offended' (p. 15). However, the acceptance of the social and personal consequences of a homicide offence can be particularly difficult to bear. This may be one reason that such groups were not offered in the past and why we met such resistance when we set up the first group. One consultant forensic psychiatrist said, 'We haven't needed a group like this for 150 years and we don't need one now,' suggesting that (in this speaker's mind, at least) offenders are stuck in a historical amber in which no change is possible to think about. When a similar homicide group was proposed for women, another psychiatrist said, 'You might as well set up a wearing-pink-bows group.' One can only imagine the level of anxiety that would generate such an incoherent statement, in which the speaker equates homicide with wearing pink.

Some of the institutional anxiety may arise from an accurate perception of the enormity of the trauma that is associated with killing a family member or partner. There is good evidence that a sub-group of these patients will experience the homicide as a traumatic event and suffer post-traumatic distress (Crisford, Dare, and Evangeli, 2008). This is especially true if the killing takes place in a grotesque or socially unacceptable way, such as military atrocities (Haley, 1974), or if the victim is psychologically important to the perpetrator (Papanastassiou, Waldron, Boyle, & Chesterman, 2004). Perpetrators of homicide can develop post traumatic stress disorder (PTSD), pathological grief and clinical depression in relation to their offences, and group therapists need to be alive to these diagnoses and the need for treatment for these conditions.

Most information on the psychological needs of those traumatised and bereaved by homicide comes from the study of secondary victims of homicide, i.e. parents, partners, siblings and children of those who have been killed (e.g. Paterson, Dunn, Chaston, & Malone, 2006). Rynearson (2001) describes the reactions of family members to a violent death, and suggests that a particular problem for survivors is that their story is an incoherent one, that cannot contain the simultaneous drama of killing and caring. He describes three phases of the distress response in those traumatised by a violent death. The first response is avoidance, where the death is acknowledged but grief and distress are denied. This is then followed by a conflict between trauma distress, which is associated with intrusive re-enactment fantasies and fear, and separation distress, which is associated with longing and searching. Rynearson describes the value of group therapy for those bereaved by homicide, emphasising the traditional group benefits of universality, altruism, vicarious learning and cohesiveness for people who are both grieving and frightened.

Studies of those bereaved by homicide do not include perpetrators of family homicide who are also bereaved. It is therefore of interest that Brunning (1982) comments on the similar psychological responses in men who killed someone close to them. He also reports that the men went through an initial stage of disbelief, reliving the trial 'in the manner of the bereaved who go through repeated circumstantial accounts' (p. 8). He also described a denial phase, where the victim is thought of as being still alive and a depressive phase characterised by social withdrawal and an unwillingness to identify with other prisoners.

He found that cohesiveness was stronger in this group than in other groups he had conducted, although it was slower to develop, and this was our experience also.

Hillbrand and Young (2004, 2008) describe therapy groups for people who had killed a parent when mentally ill. They have described how their groups enabled group members to benefit from the installation of hope. They also describe meaningful group-mediated change in their groups, especially a reduction in feelings of alienation. This reduction in alienation is an aspect of 'universality', which is said to be therapeutic (Yalom & Leszcz 2005) because it allows people to connect with others and feel they have something in common. It seems likely that people who have killed do feel profoundly alienated from others (which may be one of the factors contributing to the increased suicide rate); it is of interest that Hillbrand and Young's group members felt less alienated by belonging to a group, even a group which only had in common the commission of fatal violence. Klein and Schermer (2000) describe the countertransference responses of therapists working with groups of traumatised people. They described such countertransference as being on a continuum between primarily irrational personal conflict in the analyst to a sense of disruption and turmoil that would be normative and expected. What they seem to be suggesting is that therapists who work with the traumatised are likely to have experienced a resonance between the issues that arise in the work and any unresolved traumatic issues of their own. This is ordinary countertransference to some extent, but Klein and Schermer are also suggesting that therapists who work with the traumatised may experience more conscious fear and antipathy to being close to people who have survived terrible events. Compassion is not automatic, and ambivalence is common, particularly as the therapist becomes a 'witness' to recollected and re-enacted catastrophic events and so may experience 'vicarious traumatisation' and vicarious grief. They believe that the therapist has to navigate between containment through self-reflection and genuine emotional experience judiciously self-disclosed, very much in keeping with a mentalisation-based therapy model.

Both Klein and Schermer (2000) and Stanton and Simpson (2006) emphasise how essential good supervision is for such groups. This has been my experience also, and I would also argue that co-therapy is essential because of the enormity of the human challenge of listening to tales of murder, terror and sometimes hopeless grief. In the Homicide Groups, the therapists initially struggled with physical fear of the patients ('We are sitting with a group of murderers!'). Later countertransference problems have been more familiar ones in group therapy: splits between therapists, idealisation of the group process or fury with group members who seem not to care about what they have done.

Repentance and atonement are key spiritual themes in many traditional religious belief systems. We are struck by how often our patients say that they wish they could say sorry to their victims or to others; and how often they express the view that they will not be able to do so because it would be too much for others to hear. We are also aware of how much they wish to be forgiven, and how impossible that seems also. These profoundly spiritual themes are present in the group and raised by the members; we respond but do not ask proactively about these issues, chiefly because we are cautious about stepping outside our roles as therapists into something more associated with religious roles. We see ourselves as companions for these men as they walk their Via Dolorosa; companions who might help them bear their burdens but cannot take them away completely.

## Conclusion

After over 10 years of offering psychodynamic group therapy to forensic patients in secure psychiatric care, I have found no evidence for Stein and Brown's (1991) claim that the personality characteristics of forensic patients inhibit group-mediated change. It is true that not all patients can engage in reflective mentalising therapies, but this is true for all people referred for therapy, and takes us to the issue of assessment for therapy, which would require a paper in its own right. It is also true that it is hard to empirically evaluate psychodynamic groups like the Homicide Groups, but there are obvious indirect outcome indicators: namely, that men are assessed as less risky and are enabled to move on in their rehabilitation pathway successfully. Of course, psychodynamic groups like these are only a part of the total therapeutic effort that is made in secure psychiatric settings, but we are confident that it is a part that makes an important contribution to offender recovery, and which takes group members seriously as people.

I conclude with another excerpt from the Homicide Group at work. The conversation turns to change and the therapists comment that things are changing all the time, all through life. Here are some responses from the group members:

> P1: After death? Do you change after Death?
> P2: I think [my victim's] in Hell.
> P1: I think when you die that's it. no Heaven, no Hell.
> P3: They put you in the ground. if there's a heaven, where is it?
> P4: I'd like to believe that there's something after... but I don't know... I hope there is.
> (*A matter of faith?*) You have to believe in something... and it's something that you do.

## Disclosure statement

I have no known competing interest in relation to this paper.

## Acknowledgements

I would like to express my thanks to the men in that group, my co-therapists and my supervisor for permission to quote from that process.

## References

Adler, L. J., Skalina, L., & McAdams, D. (2008). The narrative reconstruction of psychotherapy and psychological health. *Psychotherapy Research*, *18*, 719–734.

Adshead, G. (2003). Three degrees of security. In F. Pffafflin & G. Adshead (Eds.), *A matter of security: Attachment theory and forensic psychiatry and psychotherapy* (pp. 147–166). London: Jessica Kingsley.

Adshead, G. (2011). The life sentence: Using a narrative approach in group psychotherapy with offenders. *Group Analysis*, *44*, 175–195.

Aiello, L., & Dunbar, R. (1993). Neocortex size, group size and the evolution of language. *Current Anthropology*, *34*, 184–193.

Allen, J., & Fonagy, P. (2006). *Handbook of mentalisation based treatments*. Chichester: Wiley.

Brunning, J. (1982). The group psychotherapy of murderers. *Prison Medical Journal*, *23*, 6–10.

Cox, M. (1976). Group psychotherapy in a secure setting. *Proceedings of the Royal Society of Medicine*, *69*, 215–220.

Crisford, H., Dare, H., & Evangeli, M. (2008). Offence-related posttraumatic stress disorder (PTSD) symptomatology and guilt in mentally disordered violent and sexual offenders. *The Journal of Forensic Psychiatry and Psychology*, *19*, 86–107.

Drennan, G., & Alred, D. (2013). Recovery in forensic mental health settings. In G. Drennan & D. Alred (Eds.), *Secure recovery: Approaches to recovery in forensic mental health settings* (pp. 1–22). London: Routledge.

Ferrito, M., Vetere, A., Adshead, G., & Moore, E. (2012). Life after homicide: Accounts of recovery and redemption of offender patients in a high security hospital – A qualitative study. *Journal of Forensic Psychiatry and Psychology*, *23*, 327–344.

Fonagy, P., & Adshead, G. (2012). How mentalisation changes the mind. *Advances in Psychiatric Treatment*, *18*, 353–362.

Foulkes, S. (1964). *Therapeutic group analysis*. London: George Allen & Unwin.

Garland, C. (1993). The lasting trauma of the concentration camps. *British Medical Journal*, *307*, 77–78.

George, C., Kaplan, N., & Main, M. (1985). *Adult attachment interview: Unpublished manual*. Berkeley, CA: University of Berkeley.

Haley, S. A. (1974). When the patient reports atrocities: Specific treatment considerations of the Vietnam veteran. *Archives of General Psychiatry*, *30*, 191–196.

Hashemi, B., Shaw, R. J., Hong, D. S., Hall, R., Nelson, K., & Steiner, H. (2008). PTSD following traumatic injury: Narratives as unconscious indicators of psychopathology. *Bulletin of the Menninger Clinic*, *72*, 179–190.

Hesse, E. (2008). The adult attachment interview. In J. Cassidy & P. Shaver (Eds.), *Handbook of attachment* (2nd ed.) (pp. 552–598). New York: Guilford.

Hillbrand, M., & Young, J. L. (2004). Group psychotherapy for parricides: The Genesis Group. *Forensische Psychiatrie und Psychotherapie Werkstattschriften*, *11*, 89–97.

Hillbrand, M., & Young, J. (2008). Instilling hope into forensic treatment: The antidote to despair and desperation. *Journal of the American Academy of Law and Psychiatry*, *36*, 90–94.

Karterud, S., & Bateman, A. W. (2012). Group therapy techniques. In A. Bateman & P. Fonagy (Eds.), *Handbook of mentalizing in mental health practice* (Chapter 4, pp. 81–105). American Psychiatric Publishing.

Klein, R. H., & Schermer, V. L. (Eds.). (2000). *Group psychotherapy for psychological trauma*. New York: Guilford Press.

Landers, J. J., Macphail, D. S., & Simpson, R. C. (1954). Group therapy in HM prison, wormwood scrubs – The application of analytical psychology. *The British Journal of Psychiatry*, *100*, 953–960.

Landman, J. (2001). The crime, punishment and ethical transformation of two radicals: Or how Katherine Power improves on Dostoevsky. In D. McAdam, R. Josselson, &

A. Lieblich (Eds.), *Turns in the road: Narrative studies of lives in transition* (pp. 35–66). Washington, DC: American Psychological Association.

Liettu, A., Mikkola, L., Säävälä, H., Räsänen, P., Joukamaa, M., & Hakko, H. (2010). Mortality rates of males who commit parricide or other violent offense against a parent. *Journal of the American Academy of Psychiatry and the Law Online, 38*, 212–220.

Mackwood, J. (1951). Group therapy in prisons. *The Howard Journal of Criminal Justice, 8*, 104–112.

Maruna, S. (2001). *Making good: How ex-convicts reform and rebuild their lives.* Washington, DC: American Psychological Association.

McAdams, D., Josselson, R., & Lieblich, A. (2001). *Turns in the road: Narrative studies of lives in transition* (pp. 35–66). Washington, DC: American psychological Association.

McAdams, D. P., & Pals, J. L. (2006). A new big five: Fundamental principles for an integrative science of personality. *American Psychologist, 61*, 204–217.

McCorkle, L. W. (1949). Group therapy in correctional institutions. *Federal Probation, 13*, 34–37.

McCorkle, L. W. (1953). The present status of group therapy in United States correctional institutions. *International Journal of Group Psychotherapy, 3*, 79–87.

National Institute for Clinical Excellence. (2009). Antisocial personality disorder: Treatment, management and prevention. CG 78. Retrieved from http://www.nice.org

Neimeyer, R. A. (2004). Fostering posttraumatic growth: A narrative elaboration. *Psychological Inquiry, 15*(1), 53–59.

O'Connor, P. (2000). *Speaking of crime: Narratives of prisoners.* Lincoln: University of Nebraska Press.

Papanastassiou, M., Waldron, G., Boyle, J., & Chesterman, L. P. (2004). Post-traumatic stress disorder in mentally ill perpetrators of homicide. *Journal of Forensic Psychiatry and Psychology, 15*, 66–75.

Paterson, A., Dunn, P., Chaston, K., & Malone, M. (2006). *In the aftermath: The support needs of those bereaved by homicide. A research report.* London: Victim Support.

Pillemer, D., Desroches, A., & Ebanks, C. (1997). Remembering the past in the present: Verb tense shifts in autobiographical memory narratives. In C. Thompson, D. Hermann, D. Bruce, D. J. Read, & D. Payne (Eds.), *Autobiographical memory: Theoretical and applied perspectives* (pp. 145–162). New York, NY: Routledge.

Presser, L. (2013). *Why we harm.* New Brunswick, NJ: Rutgers University Press.

Rynearson, E. K. (2001). *Retelling violent death.* London: Routledge.

Schwannauer, M. (2013). Attachment mentalization and reflective functioning in psychosis. In A. I. Gumley, A. Gillham, K. Taylor, & M. Schwannauer (Eds.), *Psychosis and emotion: The role of emotions in understanding psychosis, therapy and recover* (pp. 68–83). London: Routledge.

Stanton, J., & Simpson, A. I. (2006). The aftermath: Aspects of recovery described by perpetrators of maternal filicide committed in the context of severe mental illness. *Behavioral Sciences and the Law, 24*, 103–112.

Stein, E., & Brown, J. D. (1991). Group therapies in a forensic setting. *Canadian Journal of psychiatry, 36*, 718–722.

Steptoe, A., Shankar, A., Demakakos, P., & Wardle, J. (2013). Social isolation, loneliness, and all-cause mortality in older men and women. *Proceedings of the National Academy of Sciences, 110*, 5797–5801.

Sykes, G. M., & Matza, D. (1957). Techniques of neutralization: A theory of delinquency. *American Sociological Review, 22*, 664–670.

Van Staden, C. W., & Fulford, K. W. M. (2004). Changes in semantic uses of first person pronouns as possible linguistic markers of recovery in psychotherapy. *Australian and New Zealand Journal of Psychiatry*, *38*, 226–232.

Welldon, E. (1993). Forensic psychotherapy and group analysis. *Group Analysis*, *26*, 487–502.

Yalom, I., & Leszcz, M. (2005). *The theory and practice of group psychotherapy* (5th ed.). New York, NY: Basic Books.

# Can psychoanalysis help us to understand the causes and prevention of violence?

James Gilligan

*Department of Psychiatry, School of Medicine, New York University, New York, NY, USA*

As the most adequate theory of human personality yet created, including our propensity for irrational, self-defeating, and self-destructive behavior patterns, psychoanalysis is in a unique position to help us solve the most serious crisis that the human species has been confronted by at any point in its evolutionary history: the threat to its own survival that is caused by its own behavior, namely the compulsion to engage in violence on the largest scale that its technology makes possible, even when that causes the death of the self as well as of others. This continually expanding behavior pattern, which reduces even genocide to a minor footnote compared with the self-extinction of our whole species, is created not only by "apocalyptic" fundamentalism and terrorism ("suicide bombers"), but also by the increasing and only partially preventable proliferation of thermonuclear weapons to national rulers of questionable sanity, and the apparently unpreventable continuation of industrial/economic policies and practices that will, if not reversed, make our own small planet uninhabitable. What makes people place a higher value on the continuation of these behaviors than they place on their own physical survival (or that of their children)? That is the question to which this article proposes at least the beginnings of an answer: that when a person feels shamed and humiliated to a degree that threatens the survival of that fragile and vulnerable psychological construct called his "self" (or of the religious or cultural group with which his self has identified), he will eagerly sacrifice his body (and other peoples') in the attempt to, as he sees it, save his soul, i.e. his self and his self-esteem. The question then becomes: what are the social and psychological determinants of overwhelming shame and humiliation, and how can we protect people from being exposed to those conditions, or at least enhance their ability to respond to them in ways that are life-preserving rather than life-destroying?

The invention of psychoanalysis as a theory of personality, a form of psychotherapy, and a method of psychological research by Freud in the late nineteenth century has proven to be a powerful tool for facilitating the ancient injunction to 'Know thyself.' That is why it has always pained those who value the benefit this can bring to those who have access to it that there will never be enough psychoanalysts or psychotherapists to make this available to more than a tiny fraction of those who might benefit from it. The most adequate solution to that dilemma that I can imagine consists of having the flexibility to apply the insights gained from the labor- and time-intensive psychoanalyses of the few who can afford this mode of self-examination to the reform of the major social institutions and practices and cultural norms that shape the cognitive and affective development – in short, the personality development – of all those who are born into any specific social and cultural environment. These include such powerful influences on human development as our methods of child-rearing, our systems of education, health care, religion, criminal justice, and even our political and economic systems – all of which can have a powerful effect on people's character development, their self-esteem, their subjective and objective capacity to care for themselves and others, and their interpersonal relations and behavior.

These and other potent personality-shaping institutions, I am suggesting, can benefit from psychological insights gained from psychoanalysis, if those of us who practice psychoanalytic psychotherapy can have the creativity and flexibility to continually expand our knowledge base, to adapt and apply what we have learned from our intensive work with a few individuals to our major institutions and their practices, and finally, to succeed in educating both the general public and those who administer those institutions as to what we have learned.

My point is not that psychoanalysis ever has been or ever will be a panacea for whatever ails us (psychologically) – as if there ever could be such a thing – but rather, that it has given us what is by far the most adequate theory of human personality, the most powerful theoretical understanding of the workings of the psyche, and a new way of thinking about and investigating our own and other people's lives, choices and behavior that is more cognitively and emotionally powerful than any other method up to now.

We miss the point of psychoanalysis, I believe, if we see it or evaluate it merely as a means to alleviate uncomfortable psychological symptoms. Rather, it is a whole new cognitive structure within the area of the mind that has been called, from Aristotle to Kant, 'practical reason' – the aspect of mental functioning that asks and answers questions concerning what to do and how to live. Traditionally this has been seen as the realm of morality, in which these questions take the form 'how should I live?' and 'what ought I to do?' – to which the moralist provides moral answers that are called, in a religious context, 'commandments,' such as 'Thou shalt not kill,' 'Thou shalt not commit adultery,' etc. (Kant's answers to those questions, while more abstract than that, still consist of a set of moral rules or orders, called categorical imperatives.)

When asked in a psychoanalytic context, however, they are genuine questions, to which the therapist does not presume to provide answers for someone else. Rather, they are more likely to take the form (implicitly, even if not literally expressed in this form) 'How well is your strategy for living working for you, i.e. to what extent is it succeeding in enabling you to get what you want out of your life?' Since many people do not realize that they even have anything that could be called a 'strategy for living' (which in psychoanalytic terms means, for example, the patterns of self-defense, and the mechanisms of defense, by means of which they ward off, or keep unconscious, certain threatening wishes, impulses and temptations), but do realize that they have certain frustrations and other psychic pains that were what motivated them to seek help from a psychoanalytic therapist in the first place, they can usually answer, if they are being at least reasonably honest with themselves, that their strategy is not working very well, at least in some respects. And that recognition can be the catalyst for further self-exploration and self-examination in the service of discovering where their strategy for living came from, why it is not working, and what better strategy it could be replaced with, which the analyst will attempt to facilitate by, for example, noticing and exploring the instances in which the analysand starts to censor, rather than report and examine, whatever sequence of thoughts, feelings, and impulses he is experiencing.

The move from a moralistic to a psychological way of thinking typifies the difference between cognitive growth and cognitive development. Cognitive growth can be defined as the ability to come up with better and better answers to the same old questions, such as (for the moral way of thinking) 'what is justice?' But cognitive development consists of asking a whole new set of questions, after one has realized that the old ones were meaningless, unanswerable, or based on a whole set of assumptions that one no longer believes in, which cannot possibly enable us to attain knowledge with which to answer the questions it asks.

In the context of the present discussion, this would mean changing the question being asked from 'how should I live?' (which cannot be answered, since knowledge is not possible with respect to moral questions), to 'how can I live?' (i.e. 'what forces and processes sustain and maintain life, and which ones lead to death?'), which can be answered, since it is an empirical question, hypotheses concerning which can be tested by means of experience (ranging from one's personal life experience, in an ongoing analysis, to formal empirical data, on the part of those doing research). By contrast, there is in principle and by definition no conceivable moral hypothesis that could be confirmed or refuted by means of empirical data – because, among other reasons, moral commandments are not made in the form of hypothetical imperatives, they are made in the form of categorical ones. That is why they contain no more cognitive content than any other commandment, such as the military commandments to 'March!' or 'Halt!', which represent orders, not statements of knowledge.

So much for moral commandments. Moral value judgments, on the other hand, can never be anything more than definitions (which, like all definitions, are completely arbitrary) of what the speaker means by the moral categories he is defining, such as good and evil, or justice and injustice. These terms, no matter how they are defined, do not possess, and cannot possess, any more cognitive content than any other definition does. As Wittgenstein put it, definitions are merely tautologies, not statements of knowledge.

Those are among the reasons why modern psychology, of which psychoanalysis is the most powerful representative, is at the center of the three human sciences (the others being human biology, and the social sciences), which together have brought practical reason from the stage of cognitive development called philosophy – the assimilation of experience to (pure) reason, of which morality is a part, and which is incapable of acquiring knowledge, to the stage called science. Science does not merely mean knowledge – it is the only method for attaining knowledge, since it consists of the accommodation of reason to experience. That is, it consists of the constant testing and re-adjustment of theories and practices to the constantly growing body of new experiences or empirical data – clinical, experimental, and epidemiological – concerning human behavior, including the causes and prevention of life-threatening and lethal behaviors, i.e. the various forms of violence. It does this by changing the question from the moral ones, 'How should I live and what ought I to do?' to the scientific/empirical questions, 'How can I live?' or in other words, 'what forces and processes sustain and maintain life, and which ones cause death or disability?' Those are the kinds of questions that my colleagues and I have found some empirical answers to by means of clinical, experimental, and epidemiological research, all of which has been guided by applying and adapting psychoanalytic theories, methods and assumptions to the study of a range of violent behaviors including suicide, homicide, prison riots and hostage-taking, and systematic mass rapes as a military tactic in wartime.

The point of this article will be to summarize some of what we have learned so far concerning the causes and prevention of violence, the term that I will use to refer to the infliction of injuries, especially lethal injuries, on a human (whether oneself or another person) by a human. This is arguably the most important problem in public health and preventive medicine today, and it occurs in at least three different forms. First, behavioral violence, from homicide and suicide to war and genocide (the contemporary version of which has taken the form called terrorism). Now that we are in the age of thermonuclear weapons, which are increasingly in the hands of rulers of questionable sanity and rationality, we possess the ability to become the first species in evolutionary history to bring about its own extinction through its own behavior, rather than as a result of environmental changes beyond its power to control.

Secondly, structural violence, meaning the political and economic policies that create a social and economic structure that divides the population into the rich and powerful, vs. the poor and the weak, which has the effect of disproportionately killing the poor and the weak; in fact, killing far more of them than have died from all the different forms of behavioral violence put together (so far), as well as being the most powerful cause of behavioral violence, i.e. the most clearly identified cause of epidemics of homicide, suicide, war, revolution, and genocide. And thirdly, ecological violence, or climate change, which begins by killing the poor and the weak first, but which could end by killing us all, if we do not succeed in overcoming the forces that want to continue saying 'after us, the deluge (or rather, the flooding ocean, and lethal temperatures).'

In this short article I will only have space to discuss the first of these three forms of violence, but I do want to mention that all three of them, in addition to having the same ultimate consequences (mass death, potentially on an apocalyptic scale), also have the same ultimate psychological and social causes – namely, the desire to realize certain over-riding emotional and ideological goals even if those can only be reached at the cost of physical survival – as individuals, as groups, or even as a species. One of the emotional goals that motivate potentially unlimited violence is the wish to divide the population into the superior and the inferior, and to guarantee that oneself, and the group with which one identifies, will always be in a position that is superior, rather than inferior, to that of everyone else (as opposed to maximizing social, economic, and political equality) – even if that requires maximizing the amount of violence in the world, and risks or even requires the physical death of oneself or the extermination of the group with which one has identified.

For example, mass murderers, from the Kamikaze pilots in World War II to the suicide-bombers of today, have always been at extremely high risk of suicide as well as homicide (in fact, the same is true of individual murderers). Japanese soldiers were notorious for preferring death to the shame and disgrace of surrender, and many of their political and military leaders thought the Japanese nation as a whole should act according to the same values. And Hitler not only committed suicide, to avoid the shame and humiliation of being tried as a war criminal by those who had defeated him (saying he would rather be a dead Achilles than a living dog); his last order to his surviving subordinates before his death was for the complete extermination of the German people – the very nation, ostensibly, for whose sake he had started the war in the first place, and concerning whom he made the moral judgment that they deserved death because they had lost his war.

As clinicians, we have had no opportunities to study or interview Hitler himself or the Kamikaze pilots, directly and personally, so our knowledge about them is inevitably indirect and second-hand. However, mass murderers and the equivalent of suicide-bombers do exist in all too great an abundance in our prisons and jails, in our high-security mental hospitals for the 'criminally insane,' and sometimes even in our juvenile detention centers. And to an increasing degree, psychoanalytically trained therapists are availing themselves of the opportunity to work with these populations in these institutions. For example, the sub-specialty of applied psychoanalysis that is devoted to the treatment of people who engage in destructive, anti-social, and violent behavior was named 'forensic psychotherapy,' in acknowledgment of the fact that such individuals usually come to our attention through the legal system, by Estela Welldon at the Portman Clinic,[1] when she founded the International Association for Forensic Psychotherapy in 1991, together with a program designed to train and educate clinicians as to how to engage in psychotherapy with this population (Welldon, 2012). But that association, and the work it specializes in, was also inspired by the psychoanalyst Edward Glover's founding both of that clinic and of the Association for the Scientific Treatment of Crime and Violence some sixty years before that, in 1931. In the United States, Stuart Twemlow and his colleagues have created the *International Journal of Applied Psychoanalysis*, with the similar goal of finding ways to adapt and apply psychoanalytic insights and approaches to populations, and to human problems, beyond those that it could usefully address by means of traditional, conventional 'orthodox' psychoanalyses. And they are now editing the first textbook of applied psychoanalysis.

Even before the invention of thermonuclear and other weapons of mass destruction, Freud (1930) recognized with great foresight the danger to human survival caused by our propensity to engage in violent behavior, when he wrote:

> The fateful question of the human species seems to me to be whether and to what extent the cultural process developed in it will succeed in mastering the derangements of communal life caused by the human instinct of aggression and self-destruction. In this connection, perhaps the phase through which we are at this moment passing deserves special interest. Men have brought their powers of subduing the forces of nature to such a pitch that by using them they could now very easily exterminate one another to the last man. They know this – hence arises a great part of their current unrest, their dejection, their mood of apprehension. (Freud, 1930, p. 145)

I do not want to leave the impression, however, that my own decision to specialize in the study and treatment of violent criminals was the result of rationally assessing all the evidence and theories that I have just cited concerning the appropriateness of applying psychoanalysis to this subject. When I began my clinical training in psychiatry at the Harvard Medical School, I had no conscious intention at all of going nearer to anyone who was violent than I could avoid. I planned to devote my career to a reasonably conventional psychoanalytic practice. Then in the second year of my residency training, when the salary my teaching hospital was paying me was insufficient to enable me to support my family, which by that point included a wife and three children, I discovered that I could earn extra money by taking an elective rotation in something I had never heard of before, called 'Prison Psychiatry,' which would require me to spend one day a week in a local prison practicing individual and group psychotherapy with a selected group of convicted criminals.

Prior to that point in my training, I had been taught that the people who wound up in prisons were psychopaths or sociopaths, and that such people were – by definition – dishonest and would not tell me the truth; that they had no interest in introspection or self-examination; that their only motive for seeing me would be to manipulate me into supporting their ability to be paroled and released from prison; that they were, in short, untreatable. I had been taught that the reason they raped, robbed, or even killed others was because it was to their rational advantage and self-interest to do so, and that they merely lacked the internalized inhibitions against such behavior that the rest of us have. In other words, I thought they were in effect like graduates of the Harvard Business School, who had studied cost-benefit analysis and were behaving according to the same principles of rational self-interest and common sense. That implied that the only experience they would learn from was punishment, and the only effective way to teach criminals to stop harming others was to harm them even more, by punishing them more severely the more violently they behaved. It seemed reasonable to suppose that increasing the costs of their criminal behavior, while the benefits remained constant, would increase the cost-benefit ratio, and they would stop breaking the law. Neither psychiatrists nor psychoanalysts, I had been taught up to that point, should waste their time trying to treat these untreatable people; all we could do was hope that the courts would send them to prison, and that their punishments would teach them to behave themselves. As a result, I expected my experience as a prison psychotherapist to be boring and an exercise in futility. But I needed the money. So into the prison I went.

To my surprise, I found it to be the most emotionally moving experience I had had in my psychiatric training up to that point, for I found myself face to face with the depths of human tragedy on a daily basis – both the tragedies that these men had inflicted on their victims, but also the tragedies of which they themselves had been the victims. The most violent among them were the survivors of their own attempted murders, at the hands of a parent, or of the actual murders of their closest family members, often in front of their eyes. I also found the task of attempting to understand these men, to learn what could possibly motivate one human being to treat another human being in ways that we call 'inhuman,' the most intellectually and scientifically challenging mystery I had ever attempted to solve. Finally, I felt that the magnitude of the danger posed to our whole society, and indeed our whole species, by the human propensity to commit acts of horrendous violence made it the most socially important problem to which I could devote my career.

Fortunately for me, my training in working with this challenging population was conducted by an inspiring psychoanalyst who was the author of some of the first American articles on prison psychiatry, Adler (1972, 1982). I also had as a mentor another psychoanalyst, Elvin Semrad, who had introduced me to the notion that a psychoanalytic approach could enable us to understand and treat even the most deeply disturbed individuals, a population that even Freud had initially considered untreatable (though that did not stop him from realizing that psychoanalysis could in fact add to our understanding of even the severely psychotic when he chose to analyze Schreber's memoirs (Freud, 1911). As a result of my initial prison experience, I came to the conclusion that the main reason criminals had been considered untreatable was because almost no one had made a serious attempt to treat them.

One of the most widespread myths about violence is that the criminals who commit it behave the way they do because they are simply amoral and never developed a moral value system. In fact, I had never heard such a constant preoccupation with moral questions as I have since I began to sit down and talk with murderers and rapists; they can hardly talk about anything else but central moral issues such as unfairness and neglect, exploitation and abuse. They would rather die than submit to what they perceive as neglect or injustice (and these are not empty words – the death rate of those who engage in serious violence is many times higher than that of others of their age, class, caste, and sex).

The moral ideology typically expressed by those who commit criminal violence is exactly the same as conventional morality – except that the value signs are reversed, so that what is positively valued according to conventional moral and cultural values is negatively valued by the criminal personality and subculture. Where someone with a 'normal' value system (i.e. one that is socially acceptable in our culture) might typically be expected to feel guilt, the person with an 'antisocial' value system typically feels pride. In fact, I have often seen this reversal of conventional morality be so explicit as to take the form of a person's boasting (not apologizing) about how 'bad' he is, as a way of demonstrating how 'tough' he is (as in 'I'm the baddest mother-fucker you ever saw'); or even reversing the conventional symbols and rituals of religion (joining cults that worship Satan or 'Anti-Christ') or politics (idolizing Hitler and the Nazis).

Examples of these patterns can be multiplied almost ad infinitum in any prison or maximum security hospital. Charles Silberman, in *Criminal Violence, Criminal Justice* (1978, p. 387), has also noticed 'the inverted morality that often prevails: in prison, as in the ghetto, "bad" is "good," and inmates compete to see who is the "baddest" of all.' And this strategy for diminishing shame works, at least in the short run: many convicts have told me that the more violent they are, the more 'respect' they get from others – both guards and other inmates. That that is why they are violent is indicated by the fact that inmates almost invariably explain, when I ask them why they assaulted another person, that it was because 'he disrespected me' or 'he disrespected my visit [i.e. my visitor]'; and that if they are not violent under those conditions they will lose respect from others and even their own self-respect. In fact, they used the word 'disrespect' so often that they abbreviated it into the slang expression, 'he dis'ed me.' And it occurred to me that any time a word is used so often it gets abbreviated, that tells you something about how central it is to their moral and emotional vocabulary.

I concluded, from this and an endless variety of other evidence, that there is one experience that is necessary, though not sufficient, for the causation of violent behavior, in the same sense that the tubercle bacillus is necessary but not sufficient in the etiology of tuberculosis – though in the case of violence, the etiologic agent is not a bacterium, it is an emotion: the emotion of shame and humiliation. I will use the term 'shame' as a generic word for a whole family of related emotions, in the same sense that we use the word 'flower' to refer to roses, tulips, daffodils and so on. By 'shame' I mean not only humiliation, but also the feelings of being disrespected, dishonored, disgraced, demeaned, defeated, insulted, slighted, rejected, ridiculed, mocked, embarrassed, treated as inferior, unimportant, insignificant or a failure, or of 'losing face' or experiencing what psychoanalysts call narcissistic wounds and injuries.

I say that this experience is necessary but not sufficient for the production of violent behavior because all of us have experienced insults or slights, or have said or done something of which we ourselves felt ashamed, and yet most of us have never committed a significant act of violence in our lives. So clearly other preconditions have to be present before the experience of shame will cause violence.

The first that I will mention is that the intensity of the shame experienced is so intense as to overwhelm the psyche and its defense mechanisms, to the point that the individual experiences something that was described to me by almost all of the most intractably violent men with whom I worked, of which I had never heard before I entered the world of the prisons: namely, that they themselves had died, even before they started killing other people. What they meant by that was that their personality had died, their self. By which they meant that they felt dead inside, meaning numb, lifeless, empty, that they had lost the capacity to have feelings, either physical sensations or emotions, so that they would refer to themselves with terms that mean the living dead, such as vampire, zombie or robot, that they would feel that their bodies were filled with lifeless objects like straw, that their arms and legs were filled with ropes and cords rather than nerves and veins, so that they would cut themselves to see if they would bleed or have pain, in order to see if they were really alive. They would mutilate themselves as viciously as they had mutilated their victims, which means very viciously indeed, to see if they could have feelings, and would then discover that even doing that did not enable them to have feelings. They found the experience of deadness more tormenting than even pain would be, and they found it intolerable to be dead when other people were still alive, which added to their motivation to kill others. They would cut or mutilate themselves not as self-punishment or penance for the crimes they had committed, but in order to prove that they were alive, when they saw blood, or to see if they could feel pain, and were disappointed to find that they did not. They would kill other people to see if that could enable them to have feelings, and discovered that even that did not enable them to feel alive.

What caused that feeling of deadness? Almost always, these men would tell me when the 'death of their self' had occurred, and almost invariably, it was an experience of overwhelming shame and humiliation, in which they felt treated as totally unloved, disrespected, worthless, as insignificant as insects, and completely rejected, almost always by their parents, but also by other significant adults such as other relatives, teachers, and so on. Yet our language alone tells us this, if we pay attention to it. One of the words for overwhelming shame is 'mortification,' whose Latin roots mean 'to make dead.'

Another precondition that needs to be in place before shame will cause violence is the absence of the emotional capacities that keep most of us from resorting to violence no matter how humiliated we may feel – such as the ability to feel guilt and remorse over hurting others; the ability to empathize with (i.e. to feel oneself) the pain felt by others; and the capacity to love and care for others. In the violent people I worked with, all of those capacities were notable for their absence.

Freud believed that no one feels guiltier than the saints (Freud, 1930). And he was right, that was why they were saints – because they felt so guilty about causing pain or harm to anyone, even those who were guilty of the most grievous sins, even those committed against themselves. But I would add to Freud's insight the opposite observation, that no one feels more innocent than the criminals. That is why they are capable of being criminals, that they lack the capacity for the feelings of guilt and remorse that would inhibit the rest of us from ever committing the crimes that led to their being sentenced to prison.

And the reason that the criminals I have worked with lacked the capacity to love and care for others is very understandable once one understands the psychology of shame. For while we speak of shame as an emotion, it is actually the absence or deficiency of an emotion – namely, the emotion of self-love, or pride (i.e. the feeling of self-esteem, self-worth, self-respect, dignity, etc.). Now, there are only two possible sources of love for the self, namely, from others and from oneself. When both sources are failing to provide love for the self, then the self cannot emotionally afford to give any of its deficient supply of love to others. It needs to ration that all-too-limited supply for the self (which is why shame-dominated people are called 'selfish,' by those who do not understand what they are going through). For in the absence of love for the self, the self dies, as I have just described, just as the body dies in the absence of oxygen.

Another precondition that needs to be present before shame will cause violence is the absence of non-violent sources of pride and self-esteem, such as the skills and knowledge that are gained through education; a job, career, or profession that brings self-respect and respect from others; some standing and respect from one's friends, family and community; a sufficiently high position in the hierarchy of status, prestige, and honor in one's community, etc. Those who are most vulnerable to resorting to violence when they feel humiliated or slighted are lacking in almost all of the above. They are statistically far more likely to be not only uneducated but even illiterate, unemployed, poor, homeless, and members of minority groups that are singled out in our society for being treated as inferior in intelligence, morality, and overall worth (e.g. African-Americans, Latinos, native Americans, etc.).

When I was directing the mental health system in the Massachusetts prisons, we came across empirical evidence in support of this last point. We found that of all the self-help programs that were available to the prisoners, the one that was most successful in preventing recidivism, or reoffending, after they were released from prison was gaining a college degree while in prison. Over a 25-year period, not one prisoner, out of the more than 200 who had gained at least a college degree (and in some cases a master's degree) while in prison, returned for a new crime. At first, I thought we must have missed some, but a national canvass confirmed that none had been returned to any prison in the country. And we found that the state of Indiana had had the same result, as had Folsom state prison in California. Now of course nothing is 100% everywhere and forever, but many national surveys have confirmed the general finding that education, especially higher education, is the most effective single means of preventing crime and violence. (I should add that many of our 'graduates' had been sentenced to prison in the first place because they had committed murders, rapes, and other extremely serious violent crimes. They were hardly boy scouts.)

Why would this be so? Clearly, the acquisition of skills and knowledge through education is one of the most direct and successful means for increasing people's self-esteem, their self-respect, and their respect from others. So if there is any validity to the general theory of the relationship between shame and violence that I am presenting here, we would certainly expect the finding I have just mentioned – namely, that a college education would diminish both shame and violence.

One last precondition that increases the likelihood that shame will cause violence is socialization into what my colleagues and I have called the 'male role belief system.' For some 10 years, I served as the principal investigator of a violence-prevention experiment in the jails of San Francisco, in which we immersed 64 violent men at a time in therapeutic and educational programs 12 hours a day, 6 days a week, for relatively brief periods of time (less than a year, and often only two to four months, since they were not in a prison, they were in a jail, where sentences are supposed to be for less than a year).

One of the most interesting and effective of these was a therapy group in which a group of 12 to 16 men would spend two hours engaging in a second-by-second reconstruction of what had been going on in the mind of one of the men, during the time leading up to his committing the violent crime for which he had been sentenced to the jail. What these men revealed time after time was that they had divided the social world into the superior and the inferior, and that in that division, men were defined as superior and women as inferior. In addition, to be a 'real' man, one would have to be superior also to other men. But since neither men nor women like to be cast into an inferior role, this was clearly a recipe for violence. In this value system, if a woman challenged the man's superiority and refused to be submissive to him, he would no longer be a man if he allowed her to 'get away with' such 'insubordination.' Nearly half of these men were in jail because of violence toward women, almost always their intimate partners.

I was amazed to see how quickly these men got the point. They had not even been aware that they had these beliefs and assumptions until they participated in this group exercise and were asked to explain how they understood each step in the escalation of their interpersonal conflict toward an act of violence. Once they saw how absurd their own underlying beliefs were, they began to speak of themselves as having been 'brainwashed' by our whole society. And they quickly saw how their acting on these unconscious or preconscious assumptions had led to their behaving in ways that had ruined their own lives as well as the lives of women whom it turned out they actually wanted to continue to have a relationship with. They would be in tears because of their grief that they had irreversibly destroyed a relationship that they actually wanted. But that grief itself motivated them to want to teach the new inmates who were coming into the jail what they themselves had just learned. In fact, they wanted to lead these groups themselves. So we trained and supervised them, through role-playing exercises and other means, to become group therapists themselves (which might be seen as an adaptation of the various 'Twelve Step' programs such as Alcoholics Anonymous).

The results of this program were quite dramatic. Although correction officers had predicted that we would have riots from having all the men sleeping in an open space together rather than locked individually in cells, we found that the incidence of violent incidents dropped from 38 during the year before this new program was started, to one during the first month and then to zero for the next 12 months. And the rate of violent recidivism following release back into the community was 83% lower than it was in a matched control group in an ordinary jail during the first year after release (which is when most recidivism occurs), among those who had participated in it for at least (but not necessarily longer than) four months (Gilligan & Lee, 2004). This program was awarded a major national prize from the Kennedy School of Government at Harvard for 'innovations in American governance,' in a competition with some 800 innovative programs from around the country.

There are many things we can learn from this experiment, I believe, but one is that it provides evidence supporting the hypothesis that the male gender role into which men are socialized in our society is a major factor in stimulating male violence, which means most violence; and that enabling men to become aware that they do not have to judge themselves as shameful by these criteria liberates them from being vulnerable to shame for not being violent and domineering. To say this is not meant to deny that we need to include violent women as well in our studies of violence, for although they commit less violence than men overall, their victims, when they do, are disproportionately the most vulnerable members of our society, namely, children; and the women's lives also become ruined once they have committed a serious act of violence. One of the lacunae in my own experience in working with violent offenders is that I have had much less opportunity to work with women. Thankfully, however, female violence is also beginning to receive more attention, which can only help to advance our understanding beyond what it could ever be otherwise.

This brief article has only touched on about one per cent of what could be said about what we have learned from working with violent people, but I hope it is sufficient to convince the reader not only that applying psychoanalysis to the study of violence can provide a unique and indispensable resource for advancing our ability to understand and solve this increasingly important problem in our communal life, but also that opening up this population for psychoanalytic therapy and research creates an invaluable 'database' for the further growth of psychoanalysis itself, as a theory, a method of research, and a type of therapy.

## Disclosure statement

No potential conflict of interest was reported by the author.

## Note

1. The Portman Clinic is a National Health Service outpatient clinic in London, UK, that provides psychoanalytically informed treatments for violent, delinquent and perverse patients.

## References

Adler, G. (1972). Prison treatment: Past, present, future. *Psychiatric Opinion, 9*, 6–10.

Adler, G. (1982). Recent psychoanalytic contributions to the understanding and treatment of criminal behaviour. *International Journal of Offender Therapy and Comparative Criminology, 26*, 281–287.

Freud, S. (1911). Psycho-analytic notes on an autobiographical account of a case of paranoia (dementia paranoides). In J. Strachey (Ed.), *The standard edition of the complete psychological works of Sigmund Freud* (Vol. 12, pp. 1–82). London: Hogarth Press and the Institute of Psychoanalysis.

Freud, S. (1930). Civilization and its discontents. In J. Strachey (Ed.), *The Standard Edition of the Complete Psychological Works of Sigmund Freud* (Vol. 21, pp. 57–146). London: Hogarth Press and the Institute of Psychoanalysis.

Gilligan, J., & Lee, B. (2004). Beyond the prison paradigm: From provoking violence to preventing it by creating 'anti-prisons' (residential colleges and therapeutic communities). In J. Devine, J. Gilligan, K. A. Miczek, R. Shaikh, & D. Pfaff (Eds.), *Youth violence: Scientific approaches to prevention* (pp. 300–324). New York, NY: New York Academy of Sciences.

Silberman, C. E. (1978). *Criminal violence, criminal justice*. New York, NY: Random House.

Welldon, E. (2012). *Playing with dynamite: A personal approach to the psychoanalytic understanding of perversions, violence and criminality*. London: Karnac.

# Forensic follow-up care for outpatients in Germany

Markus G. Feil

*Evangelisches Hilfswerk München gemeinnützige GmbH, Munich, Germany*

Legislation has revived forensic psychotherapy for outpatients in Germany. Since 2007, in almost all 16 federal states of Germany forensic outpatient clinics have been and are being established for criminal and sex offenders who have been released from prison or secure detention under conditions imposed by the court. This paper reviews the consequences of this legislation for forensic outpatients, and will focus on some of the central organisational, institutional and social aspects that stem from the experience of the author. Although the conclusions may not be new, they require repeated reflection and well-considered political commitment.

Legislation, which came into force in April 2007, has revived forensic psychotherapy for outpatients in Germany. This legislation addressed 'the reform of supervision of conduct and amendment of the conditions governing subsequent preventive detention'. Since its introduction, in almost all 16 federal states of Germany 'forensic outpatient clinics', as defined in section 68 of the German Criminal Code, have been and are being established for criminal and sex offenders who have been released from prison or secure detention under conditions imposed by the court. The law also gave financial and institutional security to the few outpatient clinics that were previously operating under their own initiative from the secure hospitals.

This paper reviews the consequences of this legislation for forensic outpatients, and will focus on some of the central organisational, institutional and social aspects that stem from my experience as director of a forensic outpatient clinic. Although the conclusions may not be new, they require repeated reflection and well-considered political commitment.

## The amendment

Reform of the 'supervision of conduct legislation', hitherto regarded as a 'blunt sword', was intended to clarify the law on this matter. The 'resolution recommendation and report of the legal committee [of the German Parliament] (6th committee) from March 20, 2007' states:

> Supervision of conduct guarantees follow-up support of offenders (m/f) whose social rehabilitation seems to be in jeopardy for different reasons following their release from prison or secure hospitals and therefore requires a particular degree of controlled assistance and supervision in the interests of mending their ways and for the sake of security. [For this purpose], a crisis intervention tool is to be created with the help of which critical developments of the probands (m/f) could be better recognized at an earlier stage than in the past and the risks countered on time.

As a result, scientific knowledge flowed into this legal reform, particularly the idea of forensic secondary and tertiary prevention (including empirical indications of efficacy); however, the motives for controlling dangerous offenders and increasing security in the society were no less important.[1] This became apparent in the parliamentary debate before the law was adopted. On the one hand, the former Minister of Justice emphasised that the number of serious crimes (including the sexual abuse of children) had been continually declining in Germany for years, however on the other hand, the majority of the population still felt threatened and believed that criminality in Germany was steadily increasing. The Minister detailed the background (social changes, reporting in the media) of these conflicting developments:

> If we wish people in Germany not only to be safe, but also to feel safe, then we must not hide these facts. [...] supervision of conduct is particularly conducive to the care and supervision of sentenced persons [...]. In future, a larger number of instructions can be issued to them that are more differentiated. We will intensify the sentence in the event of breaches of these instructions and improve the powers of authority, in order to efficiently monitor compliance with these instructions. (Deutscher Bundestag 2007, p. 8904)

Although, the words 'care and supervision of the individual (former) offender' crop up in these statements – as in many subsequent debates of parliamentarians – the emphasis was on another very essential objective of this law: the change in 'an emotional state of society' to more subjective security. After all, the wording in the law stipulated 'forensic outpatient clinics' (section 68 Criminal Code), which had been rare institutions in Germany up to that point.

## The implementation of the law

Under German criminal law, a distinction is made between offenders who are fully responsible for their crimes, and those who are subject to diminished criminal responsibility (sections 20 and 21, German Criminal Code) and systems are organised accordingly for their confinement and their reintegration into society. Provided a suspended sentence cannot be imposed, patients who are not accountable or have diminished responsibility due to a causal mental illness or disorder are placed in special hospitals for the most part, or special wards of hospitals, in so-called 'secure psychiatric hospitals' pursuant to sections 63 and 64 of the Criminal Code. Those offenders who are fully accountable for their crimes are imprisoned in correctional facilities (the 'penal system'). In most of the federal states of Germany, the ministries of social affairs and health are responsible for the organisation of, and assume the costs for, the secure psychiatric hospitals. Prison detention is the responsibility of the Ministries of Justice. The Criminal Code applies in the whole country. The practical implementation of the legal consequences, however, is incumbent upon the federal states, which have differing legal provisions (in the form of laws which govern the prisons and the secure hospitals) and differ partially in their institutional and practical implementation. The outpatient clinics responsible for follow-up care are still, for the most part, only responsible either for psychiatric patients in the secure hospitals or for those offenders who have been released from prison. Nevertheless, the number of outpatient clinics which treat and care for both groups of individuals is increasing.

When the reform regarding the supervision of conduct was implemented in 2007, the few secure psychiatric hospitals expanded their existing outpatient services, which, up until then, had been operating as research or pilot projects under their own initiative (cf. Freese, 2003; Seifert, Schiffer, & Leygraf, 2003; Steinböck et al., 2004). Where new forensic psychiatric outpatient clinics were established, these were also affiliated to the existing clinics of the inpatient secure hospitals, their staffing and organisational structure corresponding to that of standard psychiatric clinics. Currently, there are 69 forensic outpatient clinics in Germany affiliated with secure hospitals (Freese, 2014). Over 5,400 forensic psychiatric patients were treated in these clinics in 2013 (ibid) at an average cost of just over 15 Euros per patient per day; a fraction of the expense for compulsory detention or prison-related costs. These costs are borne by departmental budgets and, to a limited extent by health insurance.

Comparable figures for forensic outpatient clinics for sentenced offenders are not yet available. This is because since 2008 the federal states have continued to take different approaches to developing the relevant institutions and organisational structures. For example, Rhineland-Palatinate operates forensic outpatient clinics as facilities of the judiciary itself. In other federal states, independent (e.g. Baden-Württemberg, Schleswig Holstein) or diaconal (Bavaria) providers operate the outpatient clinics; in Berlin or Hamburg it is the forensic university departments.[2] The justice ministries of the federal states, as the most important benefactors, have acted according to different conceptual ideas and financial possibilities, so that outpatient facilities differ in terms of financial, staffing and material resources. For example, until now very few forensic outpatient clinics of the judiciary have had social workers and/or doctors at their disposal, whereas these professionals are part of the standard personnel resources in the forensic outpatient clinics of the secure hospitals.

Other differences exist between the forensic outpatient clinics of the secure hospitals and those established in the penal system. Even though these populations have something in common clinically, primary diagnoses of mental illness clearly prevail in secure hospitals; especially schizophrenia, schizotypal and delusional disorders, as well as mental and behavioural problems caused by psychotropic substances, and learning disabilities. By contrast, in the penal system, it is personality disorders and deviant paraphilic preferences and disorders that prevail, insofar as diagnoses are (and can be) made. In most cases, the patients in forensic outpatient clinics of secure hospitals come from the clinics where they were committed and have been treated for several years. Therefore, for forensic psychiatric patients a closed treatment chain exists between the inpatient and outpatient setting. By contrast, the clientele of forensic outpatient clinics in the prison system have neither previously been imprisoned nor detained. During their incarceration, a substantial number of inmates reject all forms of care, support and treatment. Only a small number of inmates participate in a two-year social therapeutic treatment in special prison wards ('socio-therapeutic wards'). Following their release from prison and at the beginning of their outpatient supervision and treatment, the former inmates and their therapists initially get to know one another in the forensic outpatient clinics. They have little or no knowledge of one another beforehand. In all forensic outpatient clinics, the majority of clientele consists of offenders subject to treatment imposed by the Court, with usually no more than ten per cent accepting treatment of their own accord.

## The concepts

The different forensic outpatient clinics of the judiciary vary quite considerably in their ideas about both the purpose and deliver of care and support (cf. e.g. Psychotherapeutische Ambulanz der Justiz (Psychotherapeutic Outpatient Clinic of the Judiciary) Ludwigshafen, 2014; Verein Bewährungshilfe (Association for Probationary Services) Stuttgart, 2002). Thus, the conceptual frameworks used vary similarly. This becomes clear if one considers the terminologies of treatment methods: variously termed 'psychotherapy', 'sexual therapy', 'behavioural therapy', 'criminal therapy' and 'risk management'. Treatment is always linked to the claim of what can and is to be achieved in forensic terms. Since the objective and rationale of the treatment imposed by the court is always to diminish or control the risk of (serious) recidivism, and not to improve, let alone heal the emotional state of the patient, treatment is not considered as solely a therapeutic process. The forensic outpatient clinics in which treatments are now carried out have emerged as a result of the political will of the legislator and the government bodies that enact legislation; they are also financially dependent on them. The law is applied by prosecutors and courts that are consulted to by correctional facilities, experts, the police, forensic outpatient clinics and probation services. Consequently, a number of different people are involved in shaping the application of the law. In this context, many differing interests are at play; and each person or organisation somehow has to agree with the others involved, moving between 'care', 'support', 'therapy', 'treatment', 'control', 'monitoring', 'management' and 'prevention'.

## Individual, professional and social areas of conflict and their interconnection

Forensic psychotherapy thus takes place in an extremely tense environment; it is interspersed with individual, professional and social conflicts. For the most part, the focus is on using psychometric instruments both to assess the offenders' or patients' risk, and, less frequently, their diagnoses. Therapeutic reflection or consideration of social concerns and general conditions is rare or non-existent. Although the concern to prevent re-offending from a societal perspective seems objective and rational, it becomes very difficult for the therapist to maintain a therapeutic approach when implementing the conceptual ideas and guidelines. I will outline some of the factors which influence forensic psychotherapists (not only in Germany) and the difficulties they have to negotiate, based on a few subjectively selected examples and priorities.

The majority of offenders and patients who are bound to forensic outpatient clinics are subject to treatment orders imposed by the court within the context of supervision of conduct and probation supervision. My own evaluation of the population of sexual offenders sent to my facility, and from conversations with colleagues from other related facilities, suggests that the decisions behind these treatment orders are primarily derived from political logic rather than scientific evidence (Feil, 2011). Accurate assessments concerning the risk of recidivism, its associated risk factors, and the agreed recommendations to reduce such recidivism that are in line with empirical criteria such as 'risk-need-responsivity' (RNR) principles (Andrews & Bonta, 2012), are often lacking. One of the most influential factors when recommending and imposing treatment orders for sexual offenders appears to be the (anticipated) assumption of responsibility; justification of the assessment which would be demanded by the public in the case of a serious re-offence. It seems that the anticipated public pressure sets the 'blame game' into motion. In the event of recidivism, each person involved with the offender wants to cover his or her back in advance and protect himself or herself against the accusation of not having done everything possible to prevent the re-offending behaviour. It is not unrealistic to anticipate a very formal application of section 68 Criminal Code without the legally required review of each individual case. This means that almost every person who has served a complete sentence for a sexual offence will receive a supervision of conduct and a therapy order. In the main, this also applies to offenders on probation. However, the recidivism rates of sexual offenders tell a different tale. At least 60–80% of those who have been convicted of a sexual offence on one occasion will not re-offend, even if they have received no psychotherapeutic treatment (Elz, 2001, 2002; Kröber, 2009; Nedopil, 2006).

Furthermore, treatment orders are by no means synonymous with an indication for forensic psychotherapy. This means that the forensic outpatient clinics of prisons initially have to clarify the extent to which the court instructions imposed are realisable within the scope of forensic psychotherapy. In my opinion, two difficulties have to be overcome. Firstly, assessing suitability for forensic psychotherapy under conditions of freedom, compared to those of detention, may result in a completely different recommendation from the assessing clinician. For example, the facility in which I work manages to treat a remarkable number of released offenders in psychotherapeutic settings who, during their detention, despite offers of treatment, completely rejected any discussion relating to their offence or intrapsychic factors leading up to the offence. Secondly, in forensic outpatient clinics, assessment not only concerns the offender's suitability for psychotherapy in general, but also their suitability for *forensic* psychotherapy. Therefore, it is necessary to clarify the offender's motivation and determine the existence of psychopathology that requires treatment and is treatable, as well as its interconnection with and relevance to offending behaviour (both in the past and in the future).

For this reason, the psychotherapist in a forensic outpatient clinic for released detainees is in a similar situation during the probation phase as is described in the general conditions of sections 20/21 and 63/64 of the Criminal Code – namely in the transition area between purely assessing risks, understanding expert opinions and forensic psychotherapy. Konrad has shown that the 'assessor' and 'therapist' occupy two mutually exclusive positions. In connection with the limitation of the therapist's obligation to confidentiality vis-à-vis the supervising authority, which in Germany is anchored in the law on supervision of conduct (section 68 Criminal Code), he points out the dilemma that confronts forensic psychotherapists. Therapists are manoeuvred

> [...] between the Scylla of an investigation approach, i.e. checking whether the statements of the client indicated a threat, and the Charybdis of a 'furor sanandi' because they have to strive to eliminate a supposed danger through increased therapeutic effects. In both cases, the therapeutic approach will be dropped and the required impartial attitude lost. (Konrad, 2007, p. 3)

A similar tension exists in forensic outpatient clinics. On the one hand, the therapist's need to be non-judgemental regarding the offender's actions conflicts with the desires of others involved in the (re) integration of offenders into society who repeatedly request that outpatient clinics submit risk assessments and reports about their patients. On the other hand, there is the necessity to communicate with other professionals involved in the management of the offender within the scope of the existing legal provisions (cf. section 68a Criminal Code paragraphs 7 and 8), especially with regard to securing the safe re-integration of the offender into society.

I believe that in such institutions thought should be given to separating the advisory from the therapeutic part of the work in terms of both personal and organisational. This would give individual therapists leeway for the necessary reflection of each new case, and for the handling of the often difficult dilemmas concerning disclosure and confidentiality. These dilemmas are often enacted in the transference and countertransference. For example, the therapist may feel pushed into a punitive or monitoring, rather than therapeutic, role and the therapeutic relationship may therefore be viewed as a repetition of the offender's earlier disturbed interpersonal relationships.

As far as the application of forensic psychotherapy in the outpatient arena is concerned, I question whether empirically validated treatment manuals, which have primarily been developed and tested in the inpatient arena (for a detailed overview, see Pfäfflin, 2006), can be used in the outpatient follow-up care of released offenders. Firstly, from a solely practical and organisational perspective, a manualised, closed group therapy is easier to deliver for patients in hospital or prison, than for offenders who have been released, and whose daily activities in the community, including work, may interfere with regular attendance at therapy sessions. Secondly, these manuals tend to determine the topics to be covered, which are often focused around the offence, at the expense of everyday life and the various daily problems that emerge in conditions of freedom. This raises questions about the suitability and relevance of the content of the modules in these treatment manuals. Drawing on the results of meta-analyses of the efficacy of treatment programmes for sex offenders, Marshall and Marshall (2011), for example, no longer regard focusing on the offence as effective, but instead emphasise a positive, strength-based approach. Bateman and Fonagy (2008) question the type and efficiency of empathy training that is usually considered necessary in manuals dealing with the treatment of antisocial offenders. They claim that in therapy antisocial patients are better helped by improving their capacity for mentalisation of their own minds, especially in stressful situations, rather than primarily trying to help them foster empathy, i.e. understanding and entering into the feelings of others. Based on their empirical study of sexual offenders, Buchholz, Lamott, and Mörtl (2008) propose that rather than lacking empathy, these individuals hold a disturbed system of values and thinking that, under certain stressful emotional states or situations, negates the existence or relevance of the other person. In addition, these authors criticise the way treatment manuals are evaluated for criminal offenders as the evaluation takes place almost exclusively by means of quantitative statistical outcome research. In psychotherapy research, however, outcome and process research should not be carried out independently of one another, otherwise treatment techniques cannot be evaluated.

Empirical studies of the application of psychodynamic approaches for the treatment of criminal offenders in the outpatient setting (cf. e.g. Morgan & Ruszczynski, 2007; Lackinger, Dammann, & Wittmann, 2008; Woods & Williams, 2014) are for the most part lacking. Two exceptions are the studies of Schorsch, Galedary, Haag, Hauch, and Lohse (1990) of an integrative methodical approach, and the evaluation of Eher, Lackinger, Frühwald, and Frottier (2006/2008) for the application of transference-focused psychotherapy in the treatment of offenders. A promising new approach that will be evaluated is MBT for patients with antisocial personality disorders (Bateman & Fonagy, 2008; McGauley, Yakeley, Williams, & Bateman, 2011).

In my opinion, the exclusive consideration of patient variables, at the expense of reflecting on the therapist's own conflicts and difficulties in the therapeutic work, is insufficient in the area of forensic psychotherapy. Both Konrad (2007) and Schorsch et al. (1990) highlight the contradictions of the forensic psychotherapist's position. The more intensely the therapist becomes embroiled in his own intrapsychic conflicts, the more aggressive the offence(s) of his patients may seem, and the more these will collide with the therapist's own system of values. This makes it difficult to maintain one's own professionalism and professional loyalty towards the patient. Motivation is therefore no longer to be understood as solely an intrapsychic variable of the patient. If the psychodynamic concepts of defence and resistance are included, motivation may be understood as an interactional product of both participants in the endeavour (patient and therapist). Other authors have described similar difficulties. Heltzel (2007) showed how, in forensic psychotherapies, therapists' own destructive elements and those of whole teams can be activated and may result in 'destructive readiness of professionals to take action in secure hospitals'. Gordon and Kirtchuk (2008) reflect on how psychic elements of forensic patients are projected into therapists, in the relationships with them and into entire institutional settings. Therefore, problems and complications concerning the treatment should not exclusively be attributed to the patient. Forensic therapists, like institutions, are constantly in contact with their colleagues or patients in a precarious 'psychic' situation similar to that of the patient. If reflection, supervision and guidance is lacking on all levels, including at the institutional level (Heltzel, 2007; Ruszczynski, 2008), this can result in tremendous damage for the patients, the institutions concerned, the therapies and ultimately society itself.

For this reason, it should not be left exclusively up to offenders to assume responsibility for their deeds. The focus should also be on the difficulties of therapists, therapeutic institutions or institutions dealing with the offenders and ultimately entire societies to assume responsibility for their management and care. Indeed, these individuals are a product of society and continue to be a part of society despite all attempts to lock them away and exclude them.

As an expert in the legislative procedure on the reform of section 68 Criminal Code (supervision of conduct), Konrad points out how legal provisions can have a direct impact on therapeutic work in the forensic area. In conjunction with the initially planned (but not implemented) limitation of the doctor's/psychotherapist's obligation to maintain confidentiality in the context of supervision of conduct, he draws attention to the fact that

> [forensic] therapists [will] question which sanctions they can expect if a client commits crimes that could possibly have been avoided had the facts subject to secrecy been known. This will not be conducive to entering into therapy obligations vis-à-vis a highly problematic patient clientele. (Konrad, 2007, p. 3–4)

The fact that such problems are not only theoretically but also practically relevant is shown in the results of a study by Stiels-Glenn (2010) from North Rhine-Westphalia. According to this study, less than 10% of practicing therapists were willing to take on sexual offenders for outpatient psychotherapeutic treatment. I am also familiar with registered colleagues who are even unwilling to take on those forensic patients for community treatment who are less disturbed. In this respect, scarcely anything has changed in recent years since the situation described by Schorsch et al. (1990), and that one reason to account for the difficulties in establishing existing and new forensic outpatient clinics is the challenge of recruiting suitable staff.

The following finding also speaks for an almost systematic deficit in the willingness to assume responsibility, even in the forensic area. Hefendehl (2010) found that offenders who had committed sexual abuse who were motivated to change were more likely to be admitted to the therapeutically oriented prison wards available in Germany ('social therapeutic wards'). On the other hand, due to their more overt aggressive behaviour, offenders who had committed rape were rejected where contact proved difficult. In both cases, however, there was little attempt to ascertain whether there was a continuing risk and thus a need for treatment that was geared towards crime prevention. The responsibility for difficult and dangerous offenders would then be passed on by means of the instrument of outpatient follow-up care after imprisonment simply by going from the 'detention system' to the 'forensic outpatient clinic system'.

## Conclusions

McNeill, Raynor, and Trotter (2012) have shown how extensively institutions and their cultures have to be altered so that important empirically established principles of efficacy in forensic psychotherapy, such as the RNR principle, can be implemented. The psychotherapeutic profession needs to apply knowledge gained from forensic therapies to forensic institutions, in order to understand and constructively influence them (Ruszczynski, 2008; Yakeley, 2010). In addition, since it is no longer just the forensic clinics, prisons and their outpatient clinics that are commissioned and concerned with the re-socialisation of offenders, but increasingly 'social agencies' such as politicians, the judiciary, police forces, residential hostels, etc., each of these individuals and institutions needs to step up their research and development.

We also have to address other critical research questions within our own profession. For example, the therapist's duty of confidentiality is considered absolute by some psychoanalytic thinkers (Yakeley, 2010). This applies to forensic psychotherapies as well (Kemper, Fegert, & Fangerau, 2010; p. 460). However, such an absolute stance may be unrealistic due to contradicting legal provisions and also for ethical reasons (cf. Feil, 2012; Yakeley, 2010). Forensic outpatient clinics as institutions could play a very practical role in the coordination and facilitation of the many institutions involved in monitoring and supporting the re-socialisation process of offenders. They could do this by introducing a psychodynamic understanding of the offender and his rehabilitation, including a psychodynamic perspective on risk assessment and management. Not every offender will require forensic psychotherapy for his re-socialisation and addressing the offender's general psychosocial needs, as well as providing social skills, educational and vocational training, are also prognostically important (Kröber, 2009).

Finally, forensic psychotherapists and institutions, especially psychodynamically oriented ones, have to be open to empirical exploration and to present proof of their efficacy, safety and cost-effectiveness. Such research is expensive and requires appropriate funding in the legitimate interests of the individual and a safe society. Empirical research in the forensic field in Germany very often follows the path specified by legal provisions. Attempts are then made to find empirical criteria in the area of psychology and psychiatry for the original normative subdividing of the offender population into 'patients/madmen' and 'good/bad'. By contrast, exploration of therapeutic and prognostic factors and long-term outcomes seldom occurs. If one remains in the legal-normative area with respect to these psychopathological and prognostic questions, this type of research runs the risk of becoming normative itself. Such research could perpetuate social defence mechanisms (Menzies-Lyth, 1988), which might consist of wanting to 'solve' the issue of 'dangerousness' through its apparent objectification of an 'even better' classification of social subsystems (in this case: secure hospitals or prison). This would lead to concealing rather than emphasising the fact that criminality, delinquency and deviance are also produced by society and are therefore ultimately concerns that affect society as a whole.

I am of the opinion that new responses in terms of society as a whole are necessary in dealing with criminality, delinquency and deviance. Firstly, it would be helpful to ask the following questions: Why is so much emotionality focused on 'sexual offenders' who are a heterogeneous group of people (Kröber, 2009)? Is society divided into 'only good' risks such as those which arise from road traffic or nuclear power, etc. and 'only bad' risks such as the re-socialisation of offenders, in order to control fears that are perhaps associated with increasingly complex circumstances? Criminals and sexual offenders contribute only a fraction of police crime statistics and in Germany, the number of sexual offences in particular has declined by 25% in the last ten years. At the same time, there is no doubt that many criminal and sexual offences cause immense social, psychological and material damage. Other offences (such as burglary) also cause huge social and psychological problems and have much higher rates of recidivism. These offenders likewise show a great need for psychosocial support and, by contrast, are neglected in terms of both research as well as treatment (Kitzberger, 2013). Finally, offences classified as white-collar criminality attract very little attention.

Dartington (2010) questioned why social systems for health and social care are divided, despite scientific evidence, when dealing with those who suffer from dementia. His central response is that western performance-oriented societies ward off fears of vulnerability and long-term dependence in this way. The question is whether such structured societies will be successful in consistently considering delinquents and deviants as vulnerable groups of persons and taking care of them accordingly. This group of people is at the mercy of the 'risk of abuse by prescribed over-regulation under criminal jurisdiction, and a misconception of averting risks at the expense of granting individual freedoms' (Freese, 2014, p. 144). This group of individuals also has to be protected against both unnecessary medication and an 'overdosage of medication' in keeping with the principle 'primum non nocere' (first and foremost, do no harm).

In this respect, it is interesting to observe whether the high occupancy figures of the previous years and length of stay in secure hospitals (Kammeier, 2014) have decreased through the establishment of forensic outpatient clinics. At the moment, this is not the case. Nonetheless, the number of patients who are treated in forensic outpatient clinics has been rising since their establishment (Baur & Kinzig, 2015; Freese, 2014). The positive effect on cost/benefit of forensic outpatient clinics compared to the costs incurred for confining or imprisoning offenders is not yet apparent.

Establishing and encouraging forensic follow-up care through forensic outpatient clinics, as developed in Germany for the last seven years, is a positive approach. Nevertheless, I suggest that one must retain a sceptical attitude in supporting the development of these outpatient clinics as social agencies. The risk is that these forensic clinics uncritically assume the ideas of control and supervision for improving safety in the population; ideas that dominate in the public statements of politicians and society. In doing so, they 'forget' the fundamental standards and principles of their own profession, namely making change possible with therapeutic and other supportive means. In this case, their professionalism is in jeopardy of being perverted.

Laws and their amendments 'remind' society and its (forensic) psychotherapists repeatedly of their own standards and responsibilities. In the course of legislation adopted by the European Court of Human Rights, the provisions for subsequent preventive detention, which are established in the same law governing forensic outpatient clinics, have become obsolete (decision of the European Court of Human Rights (ECHR) from 17 December 2009; file No. 19359/049 'Mücke vs. Deutschland', NJW 2010, p. 2496 et seqq.). Subsequent preventive detention, i.e. the extension of the limited prison sentence to long-term detention of offenders still considered dangerous had to be completely re-examined in the wake of this ECHR decision. The evaluation of the supervision of conduct is therefore interesting, because in Germany the process of evaluating amended legislation rarely occurs. The relatively new legislation and legal practice of supervision of conduct was evaluated under a legal perspective (Baur & Kinzig, 2015). As a result of their empirical findings, Baur and Kinzig (2015) stressed the importance of forensic outpatient clinics within the system of forensic rehabilitation and, from a criminological point of view, made some important legal recommendations. However, their task did not consist of demonstrating the unique contribution of the (psychodynamic) forensic psychotherapy approach. Further studies are needed to examine the subject.

## Disclosure statement

No potential conflict of interest was reported by the author.

## Notes

1. The quotations and principles for these and many of the following statements can be tracked and are accessible in the online archives of the German Parliament (Deutscher Bundestag, 2007). The legislative procedure on the reform of section 68 Criminal Code incl. all expert opinions is documented there under the file reference BT-Drs. 16/1993.
2. Examples and initial information to be found at the following Internet addresses: http://www.mjv.rlp.de/Justizvollzug/Psychotherapeutische-Ambulanzen-der-Justiz/; http://www.bewaehrungshilfe-stuttgart.de/content/119/psychotherapeut-ambulanz; http://www.packhaus-kiel.de/; http://www.stadtmission-nuernberg.de/straffaelligenhilfe/psychotherapeutische-fachambulanz/; http://www.uke.de/institute/sexualforschung/

## References

Andrews, D., & Bonta, J. (2012). Viewing assessment and rehabilitation through the lens of the risk-needs-responsivity-model. In F. McNeill, P. Raynor, & C. Trotter (Eds.), *Offender supervision: New directions in theory, research and practice* (pp. 19–40). Cullompton: Willan Publishing.

Bateman, A. W., & Fonagy, P. (2008). Comorbid antisocial and borderline personality disorders: Mentalization-based treatment. *Journal of Clinical Psychology, 64*, 181–194.

Baur, A., & Kinzig, J. (Eds.). (2015). *Die reformierte Führungsaufsicht. Ergebnisse einer bundesweiten Evaluation* [Supervision of conduct after its reform. Results of a federal evaluation]. Tübingen: Mohr Siebeck.

Buchholz, M. B., Lamott, F., & Mörtl, K. (2008). *Tat-Sachen: Narrative von Sexualstraftätern*. Gießen: Psychosozial-Verlag.

Dartington, T. (2010). *Managing vulnerability: The underlying dynamics of systems of care*. London: Karnac Books.

Deutscher Bundestag. (2007). *Deutscher Bundestag. Stenographischer Bericht* 88. Sitzung. Berlin, Donnerstag den 22. März 2007.

Eher, R., Lackinger, F., Frühwald, S., & Frottier, P. (2006/2008). Beziehungsorientierte Psychotherapie bei entlassenen Straftätern und einer Gruppe von Sexualstraftätern – Ergebnisse einer 7-Jahres-Katamnese. In F. Lackinger, G. Dammann, & B. Wittmann (Eds.), *Psychodynamische Psychotherapie bei Delinquenz: Praxis der Übertragungsfokussierten Psychotherapie* (pp. 416–428). Stuttgart: Schattauer.

Elz, J. (2001). *Legalbewährung und kriminelle Karrieren von Sexualstraftätern: Sexuelle Missbrauchsdelikte*. Schriftenreihe der Kriminologischen Zentralstelle e.V., 33. Wiesbaden: KrimZ. ISBN: 978-3-926371-52-2. http://www.krimz.de/en/

Elz, J. (2002). *Legalbewährung und kriminelle Karrieren von Sexualstraftätern. Sexuelle Gewaltdelikte*. Schriftenreihe der Kriminologischen Zentralstelle e.V., 34. Wiesbaden: KrimZ. ISBN: 978-3-926371-53-9. http://www.krimz.de/en/

Feil, M. G. (2011). Führungsaufsicht und Therapieweisung bei Sexualstraftätern – Erfahrungen der Psychotherapeutischen Fachambulanz für Sexualstraftäter München. *Forensische Psychiatrie und Psychotherapie – Werkstattschriften, 18*, 53–61. ISSN: 0945-2540

Feil, M. G. (2012). Zwischen Scylla und Charybdis. Vertraulichkeit in der forensischen Psychotherapie. *Recht & Psychiatrie, 2012*, 191–196.

Freese, R. (2003). *Ambulante Versorgung psychisch kranker Straftäter*. Lengerich: Pabst Science Publishers.

Freese, R. (2014). Zum Stand der forensischen und forensisch-psychiatrischen Nachsorge in der Bundesrepublik Deutschland (Daten aus der sog. Pfingstabfrage 2013). *Forensische Psychiatrie, Psychologie, Kriminologie, 8*, 137–144.

Gordon, J., & Kirtchuk, G. (2008). *Psychic assaults and frightened clinicians: Countertransference in forensic settings*. London: Karnac Books.

Hefendehl, R. (2010). Sozialtherapie: Was der Gesetzgeber wollte und die Praxis macht. Erste Ergebnisse aus einem kriminologischen Forschungsprojekt. *Monatsschrift für Kriminologie und Strafrechtsreform, 93*, 24–41.

Heltzel, R. (2007). Die destruktiven Bereitschaften der Professionellen im Maßregelvollzug – am Beispiel der Behandlung von Sexualstraftätern. *Recht & Psychiatrie, 25*, 10–16.

Kammeier, H. (2014). Reform der psychiatrischen Maßregel nach § 63 StGB. *Forensische Psychiatrie und Psychotherapie - Werkstattschriften, 21*, 8–50. ISSN: 0945-2540

Kemper, A., Fegert J. M., & Fangerau, H. (2010). Bruch der ärztlichen Schweigepflicht bei Androhung von Gewalt- und Sexualstraftaten? Ethische und rechtliche Grundsätze als Wegweiser. *Nervenheilkunde, 2014*, 460–464. ISSN: 0722-1541

Kitzberger, M. (2013). *Einbruchdiebstahl und Legalbewährung: Eine qualitativ-empirische Studie*. Wien: Neuer Wissenschaftlicher Verlag.

Konrad, N. (2007). Schriftliche Stellungnahme zu *BT-Drs. 16/1993*. [See Note 1 and Deutscher Bundestag (2007).]

Kröber, H.-L. (2009). Kriminalprognose bei Sexualstraftätern. *Psychotherapeut, 54*, 237–244. doi:10.1007/s00278-009-0676-4

Lackinger, F., Dammann, G., & Wittmann, B. (Eds.). (2008). *Psychodynamische Psychotherapie bei Delinquenz: Praxis der Übertragungsfokussierten Psychotherapie*. Stuttgart: Schattauer.

Marshall, W. L., & Marshall, L. E. (2011). The Future of Sexual Offender Treatment Programs. In D. P. Boer, R. Eher, A. C. Craig, M. H. Miner, & F. Pfäfflin (Eds.), *International perspectives on the assessment and treatment of sexual offenders: Theory, practice and research* (pp. 683–703). Washington, DC: American Psychological Association.

Menzies-Lyth, I. (1988). The Functioning of social systems as a defence against anxiety. In I. Menzies-Lyth (Ed.), *Containing anxiety in institutions: Selected essays*, Vol. 1 (pp. 439–462). London: Free Association Books.

McGauley, G., Yakeley, J., Williams, A., & Bateman, A. (2011). Attachment, mentalization and antisocial personality disorder: The possible contribution of mentalization-based treatment. *European Journal of Psychotherapy and Counselling, 13*(4), 1–22.

McNeill, F., Raynor, P., & Trotter, C. (Eds.). (2012). *Offender supervision. New directions in theory, research and practice* (2 Aufl.). New York, NY: Routledge.

Morgan, D., & Ruszczynski, S. (Eds.). (2007). *Lectures on violence, perversion and delinquency*. London: Karnac Books.

Nedopil, N. (2006). *Prognosen in der Forensischen Psychiatrie: Ein Handbuch für die Praxis*. Lengerich: Pabst.

Pfäfflin, F. (2006). Spezielle Therapieformen. In H.-L. Kröber, D. Dölling, N. Leygraf, & H. Sass (Eds.), *Handbuch der Forensischen Psychiatrie. Band 3: Psychiatrische Kriminalprognose und Kriminaltherapie*, (pp. S349–S368). Darmstadt: Steinkopff.

Psychotherapeutische Ambulanz der Justiz Ludwigshafen. (2014). *Konzeption*. Verfügbar unter September 19, 2014, http://www.mjv.rlp.de/Justizvollzug/JVA-Ludwigshafen/Psychotherapeutische-Ambulanz-der-Justiz/Konzeption/.

Ruszczynski, S. (2008). Thoughts from consulting in secure settings: Do forensic institutions need psychotherapy. In G. Kirtchuk & J. Gordon (Eds.), *Psychic assaults and frightened clinicians: Countertransference in forensic settings* (pp. 85–95). London: Karnac.

Schorsch, E., Galedary, G., Haag, A., Hauch, M., & Lohse, H. (1990). *Sex offenders: Dynamics and psychotherapeutic strategies*. Berlin: Springer.

Seifert, D., Schiffer, B., & Leygraf, N. (2003). Plädoyer für eine forensische Nachsorge. Ergebnis-se einer Evaluation forensischer Ambulanzen im Rheinland. *Psychiatrische Praxis, 30*, 235–241.

Steinböck, H., Groß, G., Nedopil, N., Stübner, S., Tiltscher, E., von Vopelius, G., & Werner, M. (2004). Ambulante Betreuung forensischer Patienten – vom Modell zur Institution. *Recht & Psychiatrie, 22*, 199–207.

Stiels-Glenn, M. (2010). Zur ambulanten psychotherapeutischen Versorgung pädosexueller Patienten. *Recht & Psychiatrie, 28*, 74–80.

Verein Bewährungshilfe Stuttgart. (2002). *Psychotherapeutische Ambulanz*. Verfügbar unter September 19, 2014, http://www.bewaehrungshilfe-stuttgart.de/content/119/psychotherapeut-ambulanz.

Woods, J., & Williams, A. (Eds.). (2014). *Forensic group psychotherapy: The portman clinic approach*. London: Karnac Books.

Yakeley, J. (2010). *Working with violence: A contemporary psychoanalytic approach*. Basingstoke: Palgrave Macmillan.

# Creating mother and baby therapy groups in prison: emotional valuation

Pamela Windham Stewart

*HMP Bronzefield and HMP Holloway, London, UK*

Mothers in prison are at high risk of depression and other mental health issues and yet access to therapeutic services is limited. This paper describes the development by the author of two prison therapy groups: one for pregnant women, the other for mothers and their babies. Called the 'Born Inside' project, both groups are currently held in Bronzefield Prison, Surrey. The theory and principles behind the project are discussed, as well as the processes and practicalities involved in providing the therapy and specialised support to the women and their vulnerable infants. In addition, principles of forensic psychotherapy in relation to this specific prison population are described, and the situational and emotional challenges faced are illustrated through narratives of group members.

> Two traits are essential in the criminal: boundless egoism and a strong destructive impulse. Common to both of these, and a necessary condition for their expression, is the absence of love, the lack of an emotional valuation of human objects.
>
> – Sigmund Freud, *Dostoevsky and Parricide*, 1928, p. 178

In 2002, I set up a weekly therapy project called 'Born Inside' for the 12 mothers and their babies (from birth to nine months) at HMP Holloway, which at that time was the largest women's prison in Europe. The thinking behind the group evolved from my observational study of mothers and babies in HMP Holloway. Given that a significant number of mothers in prison have identified depression (30%), very few receive treatment or have had access to treatment in the community before coming to prison (Birmingham, Coulson, Mullee, Kamal, & Gregoire, 2006). Also underpinning the observational study was a question: How well would mothers be able to think about their babies, and provide them with emotional valuation, in a prison? I assumed and expected to find prison to be a place of enormous anxiety, which I imagined would impact on the mother's capacity to hold the baby in mind.

Although the HMP Holloway mother and baby unit (MBU) closed in October 2013, I had also initiated a mother and baby group at HMP Bronzefield, Surrey, in 2007, which is still ongoing. In 2004, I added a weekly group for pregnant women at both prisons. I developed this group in order to make contact with women before the birth of their babies, to encourage thinking about the baby before it is born, and to make a connection with women during pregnancy and before many of them transferred to the MBU after the birth of their baby.

This paper describes the two weekly therapy groups, now held only in HMP Bronzefield. Until 2012, I ran these two weekly groups on my own. The two groups are not funded by the prison, but by the Born Inside project.

In addition to the MBU at HMP Bronzefield, there are currently five other units in the UK: Eastwood Park in Gloucestershire, Styal in Cheshire, New Hall in Yorkshire and Peterborough in Cambridgeshire. Many women are sent to prisons far from home and family (Stephenson & Lindley, 2014). As the Corston Report (2007) into the female prison estate points out, the prison location presents problems for many prisoners' families. One of the main aids to reducing reoffending is contact with families, and yet this is hindered by the distances families must travel to see mothers, daughters or sisters. HMP Bronzefield is 40 km (25 miles) from central London and can be reached by car or rail – both expensive options for many families.

Imprisoning women differs from incarcerating men because, typically, women are the sole carers for their children, with many also having to provide care for elderly relatives. Although women make up only a small percentage of the total UK prison population (approximately 5%), of the 200,000 children who have an imprisoned parent, 18,000 have a mother in prison.

## The Born Inside project

When a woman comes to prison pregnant or has a small baby, the complexity of incarceration increases. Many mothers on the MBU speak of visiting a parent in prison as a child. Part of the thinking behind the Born Inside project is to see whether, with therapeutic support, the cycle of imprisonment can be broken or, as Joan Didion says in her novel, *Run River*, 'if the sum of all the choices that have gone before' can change (1963).

Over the years, the Born Inside project has received funding from many sources. Currently, the International Montessori Association provides the funds for an early year's specialist and National Childbirth trainer, Beverley Maragh, who assists as the project's co-facilitator.

### *The context: the MBU*

At HMP Bronzefield, the MBU is in a modern, purpose-built block separated by high walls from the main prison. The unit has a self-contained area of 12 cells, a crèche, a kitchen, administrative offices, bathing facilities, a large garden and an association/sitting room. The cells have a bed for the mother and a cot for the baby. The narrow, airless windows do not open. The cells have thick metal doors, which, although never locked, hang heavily as a grim reminder to the women of where they are.

Expectant mothers and mothers already with babies up to the age of 18 months can apply for a place on a MBU, but securing a place is difficult. Applications are fraught with anxiety as the mother has to clear many hurdles before she is allocated one of the very few places available. From the prison's perspective, the paramount consideration is that the woman will not be a risk to the other babies by virtue of her sentence (for example, child abuse, extreme violence, arson, murder). One mother who was on remand for murder had a place on the MBU until she was sentenced. As soon as this happened the baby was removed from the MBU and put up for adoption.

If a woman's sentence is long and she gains a place on the MBU, it means that our relationship can continue for over two years. Establishing a relationship with a therapist during pregnancy, which continues in the mother and baby group, provides continuity and support for both mother and baby. Many women say how much it means to them to have had the time during pregnancy to get to know me and to have me there once the baby is born. New mothers greet me with a look of relief after the birth. A familiar face to a new mother usually means a great deal, particularly in prison. This continuity is a form of emotional valuing that is often a new experience for the incarcerated woman.

They speak about sharing the pregnancy and birth with someone who has come to know them as expectant mothers, not just as criminals. They often say how much they value 'talking to an old woman'. They appreciate having someone who is not their own age and comes from outside the prison regime. Many are intrigued that I am not British (I am American), and do not see me as part of the prison establishment.

The mother and baby group provides an early opportunity to work with mothers who have had broken attachments and difficult childhoods themselves exactly at the point when these experiences are in danger of being transmitted to their babies. Providing a containing, reliable weekly group allows exploration and validation of the mother's experience. Through the reverie of the group, and the help of the unit staff, over time the group offers dynamic containment in place of the rigidity of incarceration with its emphasis on punishment.

Despite the outward swagger and bravado, most pregnant women are filled with horror at finding themselves in prison and a great sense of shame that their child will be born in custody. Already a place of enormous anxiety for women, applying for one of the limited spaces on an MBU is extremely stress-provoking. The women, many already worried about children left at home, also feel guilty about having a new baby with them, should they get a place on the unit. As the Corston Report emphasises, the imprisonment of women is devastating for families left at home. Many children are effectively orphaned by their mother's incarceration. Broken relationships – not only with the mother – changes in housing, disruptions to schooling and going into care all increase the chances of the abandoned child following the mother into the criminal justice system.

In many ways, the prison system mirrors and repeats the broken relationship of the inmate's childhood. Sentences are often short and served far from home.

Relationships with therapeutic services are frequently interrupted by sudden prison transfers or changes in key prison staff (Menzies-Lyth, 1988).

Working with mothers in prison allows an insight into relationships between mothers and babies often out of reach of psychotherapy intervention in the community due to lack of services. Given their own early experience, many of the mothers are suspicious of external services, having frequently been the product of the care system themselves. One pregnant woman, Lisa, reported that she experienced 56 foster carers before finally being given a flat of her own at the age of 16: 'I was left to get on with it'. When 'Laura' received a conviction for murder, she gave up trying to maintain contact with her baby son after he was born. Worryingly, the baby was given to Laura's own mother to bring up. Finding visits with him too painful, she ceased contact with him completely.

Many psychoanalytic theorists have postulated that serious difficulties between mother and infant can have adverse consequences for emotional development. Central to psychoanalytic thinking is Winnicott's emphasis on the importance of 'good enough relationships' for a child's development: 'There is no health for the human being who has not been started off well enough by the mother' (Winnicott, 1971). By supporting the mother in the therapy group, I hope to assist her capacity to think about her own experiences and feelings, which, in turn, should help her think about her baby in a way that is more than a repetition of her own early experiences. The more playful and non-judgemental I can be with the women, the better the group proceeds.

The weekly mother and baby group is structured along the same lines as a conventional therapy group. We meet at the same time each week – a Friday afternoon – and in the same room. The group is presented to the women much like one they might choose to attend in the community. The room, pleasant and airy, has toys and cushions spread about, similar to a children's library. The prison expects the women to attend the group, but they are not punished if they do not. Sometimes the women do not attend. When a woman returns to the group we have an opportunity to explore what missing the group might mean to her and to the others. The group encourage the woman to think about the feelings underneath her behaviour and not to dismiss it through blame. The idea that behaviour has meaning and significance offers a new perspective to people hardened by punishment and blame.

### *Support and stability*

Although both the pregnant mothers and mother and baby groups aim to provide an environment of stability, the unit itself is unsettled by frequent arrivals or departures of mothers, babies and favourite staff members. Confidentiality, a cornerstone of psychotherapy groups, has to be adjusted (some might say abandoned) in a prison therapy group. When a new woman joins the group, a more established member explains the general offer of confidentiality. She says that the information that comes out of the group 'needs to remain in the group'. This is often chanted out by the other members who are veterans of groups but who continue to struggle linking rules with behaviour: a central issue for offenders. The limits of confidentiality are also discussed – disclosure of criminal plans, self-harm or risks to children must be disclosed to the prison – and the members of the group need to be reminded of this.

If a mother does make the transition from the pregnancy group to the mother and baby group, there are adjustments required between the new mother and the facilitator. This can be very difficult if the new mother has no external support in the community. This is not only the case for foreign nationals who understandably have trouble keeping family ties because of geographical distance, but also for many British women whose contact is non-existent due to family breakdown, often involving the criminal activities of their partners or own parents.

### *Coping with challenging emotions*

Being in any group requires a level of maturity that arises from the capacity to have relationships. One challenge of running a prison group is that this capacity is exactly the difficulty that propels women into prison in the first place. Groups generate primitive anxieties, always close to the surface but even more so in prison. Given the high percentage of sexual abuse the women have suffered, their broken relationships and own experience as children of 'bad enough mothering', many prisoners find being alone in a room with others extremely threatening at the best of times, never mind during the emotional and hormonal upheavals of pregnancy and birth.

As the facilitator, it is essential that when it arises, the women's anxiety is given straightforward acknowledgement. This also provides them with a language to use for further reflection. For example, reflecting back to the mother that she sounds deeply unhappy or furious works. However, the question 'How does that make you feel?' is best rephrased, as it is usually met with derision and is based on the, often false, assumption that the mother has words for her feelings. A difficulty for offenders is the absence of emotional, descriptive language, which leads to actions instead of thoughts (Campbell, 2005).

When Alice stood up, ready to storm out of the group, I was able to suggest that perhaps if she could just stay in the room with us we could try to figure out together how she was feeling. She said: 'That's my problem. When I get pissed off I just run away and nothing gets sorted. I guess you are just being patient with me'. Then she sat down. Working with Alice during her pregnancy when she was detoxing established a trusting relationship between us by the time her daughter was born. When her very frail baby arrived, Alice found it very difficult to put her on the floor or encourage the baby, as she grew older, to explore independently. Gradually, as Alice gained confidence from the group, both mother and baby became freer in the use of the space. Initially wary of women in general,

Alice, upon release from prison, expressed her gratitude for the support she had felt from both groups.

### *Keeping thinking alive*

Sitting on the floor with the mothers, the group is not always able to maintain the circle symbolic of the mother's arms. At a premium in prison, adequate space is essential for the group, but often hard to find. Toddlers require space to roam if the group is to speak freely. Mothers with babies may choose to sit on chairs or join the rest of the mothers on the floor. This varies and needs to be kept flexible so there can be a sense of reliability and stability that is not strict and rigid and thus so easily identified with their experience of the prison regime. Being confronted with the high levels of anxiety and initial suspicion requires a very straightforward acknowledgement of the anger and mistrust that can be present. Keeping any thinking alive is a struggle. No one is helped by clever interpretations, which, when given, are usually lobbed back by the derision in the mothers' eyes.

Rants against the regime have to be considered and not responded to in a way that encourages splitting. Sometimes the best thing is to say as little as possible. However, easy it might be to make an interpretation that a complaint against the prison might in some way be a communication about their own mother (prison can't feed me, look after me, get me my medicine), it is usually better to acknowledge how hard it is for them being in prison and how this might make them feel about their baby.

The rants against the prison, the world and the criminal justice system represent some of the defences used against the anxiety felt by the women, and indicate a distant emotional connection with their baby. Encouraging them to imagine what their babies will be like, inside, not only in their own bodies but also with them in prison, takes time and requires trust to develop. Gradually, as the women become more reflective and curious about their baby and how it might be feeling, the baby develops in the mother's mind as a real person, and not simply a narcissistic extension of themselves (Welldon, 1992).

Being attentive and quiet is a key maternal skill useful to the therapist, no matter how much the therapist would like to relieve her own anxiety by speaking. Containing my own feelings depends on my own personal therapy and supervision. Forensic work cannot be done alone.

### Applying the basic principles of forensic psychotherapy

According to West (1996), there are two basic principles of forensic psychotherapy. The first is that the forensic psychotherapist must consider the crime as a symptom. It is extremely important for the therapist to keep in mind the mother's offence. Asking in the group is not appropriate. For one thing the mothers live with each other while the therapist is there only once a week. Very often the woman does not want to say why she is in prison and may have lied to the other women. While acknowledging that Keats's theory of 'negative capability' – the capacity to contain uncertainty 'without any irritable reaching after fact and reason' (1817) – is important in psychotherapy, there are such things as facts. These are available and necessary for the therapist working in prison. To wait until the forensic patient brings up her offence not only means that the therapist might wait forever but might indicate that the therapist has lost her bearings and has forgotten, or cannot face the complexity of the forensic setting. These are not women in the community. True, the groups are presented as something the women might actually attend in the community; however, being with the women should not be normalised in the therapist's mind as a way of minimising the destructiveness presented by the mothers. Being in a room with tender, breastfeeding mothers who have also committed serious offences can be very challenging.

Again, this is another difficult tension for the therapist to hold on to. The mothers are mothers with their babies. However, they are also in prison for specific offences that have meaning. How to hold on to the mother's experience in a non-persecutory as well as non-collusive way is a part of the struggle and requires regular supervision and care of oneself. As West writes (1996), the therapist 'is aware that too much anxiety renders him controlling and therapeutically impotent, whereas too little anxiety borders on psychopathy'.

Keeping in mind the offences while also struggling to keep the group a place of containment and thought means the therapist must maintain close relationships with the prison staff at the same time as protecting the confidentiality of the group. The therapist is with the women only once a week; the prison staff are with them all the time.

West's second principle of forensic psychotherapy is not to work in isolation, but to join with colleagues to support the therapy. This requires a respect for teamwork and personal humility. Central to running any group is respect for relationships. It is vital for the therapist to have honest relationships with the staff, who are not supported (as is the therapist) with supervision and reflective practice groups. Poor staff relationships or staff rivalry with the therapist can have catastrophic results for mothers and babies. At the end of one HMP Holloway group, I later learned an officer had been talking with the mothers asking them how they were feeling. Two of the mothers became very aggressive. With their babies in their arms, the mothers attacked each other, kicking and screaming. The babies were removed from the prison within hours. Later when I was talking with the officer about what happened, she said, 'Well, you just talk, don't you?' It is important for the therapist to remember the potential envy and competitiveness which his/her presence may stir up in staff members.

What looks simple – talking with the mothers about how they are feeling – is not without its risks. In the above case the outcome of talking resulted in the babies being permanently removed and the mothers losing their place on the MBU.

Developing relationships takes time. To meet mothers before they give birth provides a strong bond for their entry into the mother and baby group. Working with the midwives and making contact with the pregnant women helps establish a relationship that is supportive once the application for the unit is accepted and the baby is born. On a separate note, there is huge need to support women who give birth while in prison and are not allowed by Social Services to keep their babies. One woman told me that her baby had been removed by Social Services. As she walked away after we spoke, I saw she had a baby's dummy attached to her belt. This was all she had left as a reminder.

### *Curiosity about the baby*

Initially, with the pregnant women the lack of thoughts about their baby is disturbing. The longing for a boy by women who have been brutally abused by fathers and other men can make it hard to be with them in the group. When asked why the expectant mother prefers a boy, the answers are always unclear and range from having a son to protect them to not having to worry so much about boys. Men seem to be regarded more highly than women, by the women. One mother said that having given birth to a son, she now felt as if she would never have to have sex with a man again. There was a stunned silence in the group after these words were uttered. When I tried to explore further, the group remained in what felt like a very uneasy state and I did not get any further with this.

Rigid thoughts, blame and lack of curiosity are indicators of how little emotional validation the women seem to have received growing up. This leads to thinking about how little emotional validation and reverie they may have to draw on as mothers to their babies. When asked what they want for their babies, the mothers initially reply with a verbal shopping list of expensive equipment. Over time they come to speak more about being able to love and understand the baby rather than simply to dress it up. This is a poignant indication of how little they were loved and seen as individuals in their own childhood. To the women, expensive equipment equals being a good mother, until some of this can be explored. When a mother invites me into her cell to show how she has made an area for her baby to lie on the floor and move about instead of being imprisoned in a baby walker or buggy, we are able to talk in the group about ways in which maternal thinking provides an environment in which to encourage the baby to explore and to have thoughts of its own.

The mother's mind is of value, and pivotal to the emotional as well as physical development of the child. The idea that the mother's mind is important – more important than a new buggy or smart shoes – comes as a surprise to many of the women. One mother described shoplifting children's clothes so that her own children's appearance would reflect what a good mother she was. We spoke about how this thinking had led her to prison, which separated her from the very children she was attempting to care for through her thieving.

### *Sibling rivalry*

Infantile levels of anxiety provide raw material for group discussions. New arrivals in the mother and baby group challenge the group as it reconfigures. Sibling rivalries erupt not only between the younger members of the group but also for the mothers and their relationship with me. New clashes occur between the new mothers and the resident mothers. Struggles to accommodate the new baby take the attention from the older babies. Often the older babies react jealously, as in a family, making it difficult for the mothers to support, instead of punish, their baby. Recently, a new mother arrived with her three-day-old baby. The oldest baby, now 16 months, furiously began head-butting a smaller toddler, taking the group's attention away from our attempt to welcome a new member.

With the arrival of a new baby on the MBU, the older, senior babies vie for attention in the group. Having spent time on the unit and continuing to develop physically, the baby gradually becomes a toddler. Walking means more independence and a different perspective. How this increased freedom of movement, so different from being in prison, is managed by the mother brings further material for the group to experience and explore.

### *Additional challenges*

Breaks between the therapy sessions are always difficult, and Glasser's 'core complex' is particularly helpful in thinking about breaks. The forensic patient often fluctuates between longing for a 'blissful union' with the therapist and a fear of being merged with the therapist leading to a 'feeling of a permanent loss of self' (Glasser, 1979, p. 284). The group is often very unforthcoming and hostile before and after breaks. Although a great deal of time and preparation is put into working with the breaks, these are periods of regression for some mothers, who will ask for sweets and biscuits to be brought in, or there will be an increase in thumb-sucking by some of the women.

Being left behind by the therapist at the end of each group has a much greater effect on imprisoned women because not only are they being left, but they are being left inside a prison; the therapist, meanwhile, can take the keys, leave the building and go home. This freedom to move in and out of prison can be a topic of discussion in the group as it can provoke envious feelings as well as stirring up a sense of abandonment. When this was once confronted head on in the group, one of the mothers said 'but we know you will be back'.

One of the missing persons in both the pregnancy group and the mother and baby group is usually the father, who is not involved in the pregnancy. Often the father is the woman's co-defendant and also in prison. A group about becoming fathers might be very useful for some of these, often very young, men who are excluded from the process of parenthood through their imprisonment.

### *Punishment within punishment: Tracey (British Mother, convicted of theft) and her 16-month-old daughter, Chanel*

Summer arrived. The association room was awash with warm sunlight. Tracey and her daughter, Chanel, seemed relaxed and confident sitting on the floor as the group gathered. Looking around the room with a smile, Chanel babbled with confidence and speed. As her curiosity was also increasing, she headed towards one of the smaller babies who was being held by her new and slightly apprehensive mother. Looking into the sleeping baby's face, Chanel turned as if bored by it. Perhaps other mothers felt like this? This was an opportunity to talk about new babies and what was going on for them.

Catching sight of a more mobile child, Chanel headed off in his direction. Chanel tried to pull the toddler's toy away, in an attempt to engage him. As Chanel pulled the toy, her mother looked worried but said nothing. Perhaps as a result of her mother's face Chanel seemed to pull harder. Tracy called from across the room: 'Stop being so naughty.'

There was tension. The group seemed to freeze. As gently as I could, I asked Tracey what she meant by 'naughty'. I said I wondered how Chanel might be feeling with new babies in the room. What is it like when the group changes – for us, for the babies? Over the weeks Chanel's exploration increased – and so did her mother's unease.

Many feelings gathered as their date of release drew near. Mother and daughter were scheduled to return to their home in south London. Going home presents a huge transition for a baby born in prison and for the 'siblings' left behind. Chanel would be losing her first home and all the relationships she had established with the other mothers, babies and staff. A long-serving baby's departure also has a huge and often unacknowledged impact on the very dedicated crèche workers who never see the child again. The staff do not have supervision to help them manage these feelings.

Over the following weeks, Tracy dressed Chanel in increasingly elaborate and expensive clothes, as if to cover up her own ambivalent feelings to do with leaving custody. Here, we see the concrete thinking of the very anxious – if something looks lovely and sparkly, then everything is fine. Part of the validation of the group derives from challenging these certainties in ways that contain rather than increase anxiety. Despite the lovely surface, Tracy continued to struggle with Chanel's increased independence (as well as having worries of her own independence – her imminent release from prison and going home to Chanel's father).

As a group we tried to talk about how freely Chanel was moving around the room. Also we spoke about the anxieties that come as release dates approach. During the next group the following week, Tracy suddenly scooped up Chanel and placed her forcefully on a 'naughty cushion'. I expressed some surprise, saying I had not seen the cushion before. Was this something new that the mothers had been thinking about? What did the group think? We then were able to talk about what babies might learn from being punished and, in the mothers' experience, did punishment ever work? The women became animated. They were able to reflect on the paradox of mothers punishing their own babies while in a prison. We were also able to link the need to punish children in order to get rid of our own confusing feelings – particularly strong mixed feelings as great as the approaching date of release. Being able to talk about these very mixed feelings about the end of their prison sentence seemed a huge step rather than the usual one-dimensional jubilation about going home. The mood in the room shifted, becoming more thoughtful.

## Conclusion

In 2002, the New Zealand Family Help Trust published a report of its evaluation of mother and baby prison units in the USA. The research study found that mother–infant attachment was significantly greater for nursery inmates vs. the general prison population, and that there was a lower reoffending rate compared to the general prison population (Robins, 2012). However, despite these positive findings, prisons are disturbing environments and can potentially contribute to a disturbed relationship between a mother and child with catastrophic lifelong implications for both. Twelve hours a day isolated in a cell is hardly the best way to support the relationship between a mother and baby during pregnancy and the first 18 months of life.

Lacking a father or Oedipal third to take the mother away from early enmeshment puts mother and baby at risk of perverse enmeshment, as described by both Chasseguet-Smirgel (1985) and Welldon (1992). Isolation heightens the risk of perverse mothering, where the baby is potentially experienced as an extension of the mother and not as an individual with an emerging mind of its own. As Hobson describes in 'The Cradle of Thought' (2002), a baby learns to think by being thought about. Locked in a cell with the mother is not an optimum setting for this process to begin.

To provide a place for thinking about the emotional process of becoming a mother, to be alongside a woman as she becomes a mother, to hold her feelings in mind despite the physical incarceration, to validate her feelings and to encourage the growth of love – these are the thoughts underpinning both prison groups. To give the last word to Claire, a young mother: 'We never would have had this experience if we had not been in prison'.

## Acknowledgements

I would like to thank Beverley Maragh, Professor Joan Raphael, Dr Paola Franciosi and Dr Gill McGauley, as well as all the mothers and prison staff I have worked with over the years.

## Disclosure statement

No potential conflict of interest was reported by the author.

## Funding

This work was supported by the International Montessori Association.

## References

Birmingham, L., Coulson, D., Mullee, M., Kamal, M., & Gregoire, A. (2006). The mental health of women in prison mother and baby units. *The Journal of Forensic Psychiatry & Psychology, 17*, 393–404.

Campbell, D. (2005). Metaphor and the violent act. *International Journal of Psychoanalysis, 86*, 801–823.

Chasseguet-Smirgel, J. (1985). *Creativity and perversion*. London: Free Association Books.

Corsten, B. (2007). *The Corston Report: A review of women with particular vulnerabilities in the criminal justice system*. London: HM Stationery Office. Retrieved from http://www.justice.gov.uk/publications/docs/corston-report-march-2007.pdf.

Didion, J. (1963). *Run River*. New York, NY: Pocket Books [Reprinted in 1994, New York, NY: Vintage].

Freud, S. (1928). Dostoevsky and Parricide. *SE, 21*, 177–196.

Glasser, M. (1979). Some aspects of the role of aggression in the perversions. In I. Rosen (Ed.), *Sexual Deviation* (2nd ed., pp. 278–305). Oxford: Oxford University Press.

Hobson, P. (2002). *The cradle of thought: Exploring the origins of thinking*. London: Macmillan.

Menzies-Lyth, I. E. P. (1988). *Containing anxiety in institutions*. London: Free Association Books.

Robins, L. (2012). *Mother and baby prison units: An investigative study*. New Zealand: Family Help Trust. Retrieved from http://www.familyhelptrust.org.nz/images/stories/Winston_Fellowship_2011_Robins_Final.pdf.

Stephenson, M., & Lindley, B. (2014). *Mum's the word: A guide to being a good mum in prison*. London: Prison Advice and Care Trust (PACT).

Welldon, E. (1992). *Mother, Madonna, Whore: The idealisation and denigration of motherhood*. London: Karnac.

West, A. (1996). The risks of burnout. In C. Cordess & M. Cox (Eds.), *Forensic psychotherapy: Crime, psychodynamics and the offender patient, Volume II: Mainly practice* (pp. 229–240). London: Jessica Kingsley.

Winnicott, D. W. (1971). *Playing and reality*. London: Routledge.

## Further Reading

Stewart, P. (2015). A psychodynamic understanding of mothers and babies in prison. In L. Baldwin (Ed.), *Mothering Justice: Working with mothers in criminal and social justice settings*. Hampshire: Waterside Press.

Tomas-Merrills, J., & Chakraborty, A. (2010). Babies behind bars: Working with relational trauma with mothers and babies in prison. In T. Baradon (Ed.), *Relational trauma in infancy*. London: Routledge.

# A child's loss becomes a young man's violence

Carine Minne

*The Portman Clinic, Tavistock and Portman NHS Trust, London, UK*

This paper describes the contribution of earlier traumatic loss to the later violent eruptions, with fatal consequences, of two young men, one who killed his mother and one who killed an unknown woman. Their developing personalities became disordered during their disturbed childhoods and the link between these developing personality disorders and psychoses is referred to. The need for long-term treatments is emphasised, as well as the importance of communication between therapist and clinical team.

One of the striking features about working with mentally disordered patients who have been violent is the frequency with which they have experienced traumatic losses in childhood. The serious violence that erupted in the boys I have treated as teenagers appears to have been connected to an earlier traumatic loss. Indeed, in many of the patients seen in high-security hospitals, whether they are diagnosed as suffering from psychosis or personality disorder – something of an artificial divide that I'd like to return to – the degree of earlier traumatic loss is always prevalent. In other words, their breakdowns as adolescents, which takes the form of a violent enactment, has almost always been preceded by an earlier breakdown in infancy, which usually went unnoticed (Sohn, 1997). The losses can be of various kinds but the common denominator is one of loss of a consistent, reliable loving, primary object that was able to contain and process the infant's projections and to help them negotiate the sensitive and complicated developmental shifts and contained disillusionments required for gradual psychological maturing. Another way to describe this is enabling the infant to progress from the 'paranoid schizoid' position to a more 'depressive position' (Klein, 1935, 1946). Tragically, the perpetrators, the victims of their assaults, along with all the involved family and friends, also suffer from the patient-perpetrator's earlier traumas, providing potential ingredients for future disturbance in all affected in the next generation too. In that sense, trauma is 'contagious'.

I would like to describe psychoanalytic work with patients diagnosed as suffering from personality disorders who have been fatally violent to others, violent to themselves and who have a phenomenal capacity to be violent to their own and others' minds. This is in order to illustrate the impact of earlier loss traumas on subsequent development. The disturbed, and disturbing, patients seen after the catastrophic violent acting out, present psychotherapeutic challenges as they have less integrated mental structures than would generally be considered able to make use of a psychoanalytic approach (Warren, 2003). I propose that they can make significant changes with this treatment, in the context of a multi-disciplinary team care within a containing physical environment. This progress can be monitored clinically and recorded (OPD Task Force, 2008) and involves manifest changes in their mental states, shifting from a more personality disordered presentation, defending against a psychosis lurking beneath, to one more in keeping with a neurotic picture, including the development of symptoms reminiscent of a post-traumatic stress disorder. I will refer to this shift again later.

Regardless of their diagnoses, people who have carried out serious violent offences often have limited awareness of themselves and of the seriousness of what they have done. This absence or avoidance, provided by an arsenal of defenses, psychotic and non-psychotic, appears to be necessary for the patient's psychic survival. These defenses became established as an alternative to earlier mourning which was not possible in the context in which, in younger years, these children found themselves. Indeed, when they are seen later as young people, addressing their defenses can cause massive anxieties about 'cracking up' and can lead to psychotic breakdowns and, perhaps, to suicidality or even, suicide. Yet, to leave these defenses untouched can leave essential ingredients intact for being violent again. The therapist's task is a delicate and complicated one. Firstly, helping the cultivation of awareness in the person's mind without seeming to commit a violent assault to that mind. Secondly, clinically judging if and how such awareness is developing and, thirdly, continually gauging in what way that person is using this. These are reflected in the mental state changes that we look for in the monitoring of our work. It is also these shifts, or, prognostically positive internal world changes, that can provoke particular negative therapeutic responses. In some cases, the careful and limited use of anti-psychotic medication can helpfully sedate the more intense psychotic anxieties, making ongoing psychoanalytic treatment possible.

I would like to refer to how these patients are traumatized threefold because this is so relevant to working psychotherapeutically with them. Firstly, they are traumatised by their appalling background histories of losses and abuse, secondly by the offences they committed (often under-acknowledged by professionals) and thirdly, by their gradual discovery, during treatment, of having a mental disorder. This can lead to a development and manifestation, during the course of treatment, of a post-traumatic stress *type* of disorder, which should be considered a positive prognostic indicator. In other words, as awareness and understanding develops, patients begin to suffer from the consequences of this. These are the shifts that can provoke particular negative therapeutic reactions, the aims of which are to return the patient's mind to its previous disturbed but familiar state. One reason for this is that a return to oblivion is more desirable than managing the burden of awareness. I will illustrate some of what I've said with case examples. The two patients described were seen in once a week psychoanalytic psychotherapy. Some details have been disguised for the purpose of confidentiality.

### Case 1

Mr. A is now 26 years old and was admitted to a high secure hospital having been convicted of murder. Late one night, he carried out what appeared to be an impulsive unprovoked and fatal attack on a lone woman using a huge knife. Unusually for a young violent man seen in high security, he had no prior record of offences, violent or otherwise.

At first, he described his offence as a one-off event, a handbag theft that had gone wrong. However, the extreme violence used was not in keeping with this explanation and it was considered early on that psychically, a different scenario may have been acted out and after several months in treatment, it emerged.

Mr. A was the first child of married middle-class parents where father worked and mother became a full-time mother. His lasting memory of her before she gave birth to his sister when he was 3 years old was of her sitting in his bedroom as he went to sleep and seeing the red tip of her burning cigarette moving forwards and backwards and finding this comforting, knowing she was there. His mother in fact left the family home unexpectedly within a couple of weeks of his younger sister being born, leaving her husband to look after a 3 year old toddler, Mr. A and a newborn baby. Mr. A recalls his father telling him 'You know that woman who lived with us, well she's gone and she isn't coming back'. She had run off with a lover and we can only speculate as to what kind of dreadful post-partum state she may have been in at the time. The father was helped out by his own parents who lived nearby. When Mr. A was 9 years old, his father announced that a woman was moving in to live with them – his new partner, who came with her own slightly older two children. For Mr. A, this woman became the archetypal wicked stepmother. He hated her right from the start and from the information available, it sounds as if this hatred was mutual. Even before she arrived, Mr. A was already showing signs of disturbance at school. He was considered very bright but got into trouble regularly by attacking other children, usually immediately after their mothers had dropped them off at the school gate. His sister had such a bad relationship with this stepmother that after a few weeks, she left to live with paternal grandparents.

Mr. A pleaded to have therapy but then complained about how little this was compared with what he needed. The major loss, perhaps in combination with his particular constitution, may have produced unbearable feelings of rage he had to get rid of. Around the age of 4 years, he began to repeatedly draw violent pictures of people attacking each other with weapons. He also started to behave aggressively towards children who seemed to have 'nice mummies' bringing them to school. Sadly – and of course with the benefit of retrospection, he was only reprimanded at school for his naughtiness and encouraged, for example, to draw nice pictures instead.

With the onset of puberty, Mr. A's unresolved rage became attached to his developing sexual feelings. Around this time, his relationship with his stepmother deteriorated further and he constantly did the reverse of whatever she asked of him. She would then complain about him to his father who would scold him for having irritated her but neglect to explore with him what might be troubling him. He began to masturbate to fantasies of rape and strangulation. This evolved into stalking women and several times, he came close to attacking a particular woman he had been following, only to 'chicken out' at the last moment, leaving the woman totally unaware of what had nearly happened to her. By the time he was 16 years old, he was kicked out of home and ended up living in a hostel for homeless young men. He spent his days sleeping and nights wandering around aimlessly. He got money by breaking into charity shops and stealing the teddy bear for the blind or the boat for the lifeguard collections of coins. On one occasion, his hostel room was broken into by a boy living upstairs in the same hostel and some of his meagre belongings were stolen. His response to this was to break into that particular boy's room and steal that boy's prized large serrated knife, carrying it around in his pocket making him feel powerful and safe. Around this time, his sister came to spend a day with him, having had a row with the grandparents. They played in a park and went to Mc Donald's and by the time evening fell, she became anxious and they had run out of money. Mr. A took her to a police station in order to arrange for her to get home safely and the police provided her with a train ticket after making a telephone call to their grandparents. After he set her off on the train, (another more immediate loss tinged with envy) a deep feeling of rage filled Mr. A up and he got into a familiar state of wanting to stalk and attack. The poor victim was not so fortunate as her predecessors. He hung around the station after his sister left, unsure of where to go but late at night, boarded a mostly empty train. A woman was walking down the carriage as he went up it and their eyes met briefly. She turned away and started walking in the opposite direction, as though she had just changed her mind. He then proceeded to attack her with the knife, stabbing her repeatedly from behind.

What was presented by him initially to the team as a theft that went wrong could later be seen in quite a different light, an apparently impulsive attack, which was actually one that had been premeditated and rehearsed over several years. There had been an ominous development of escalation in his dangerousness from fantasy only, to practising carrying these out, and finally, an incomplete enactment of his main fantasy. Here we can see how the capacity to symbolise through the use of fantasies gradually broke down as the severity of psychotic functioning increased, leading to the need to act out. Anxiety became engendered by the very fantasies that were created in order to attempt to alleviate it. This fuelled the escalation until the fantasies no longer sufficed and a deterioration, or spillage, into action occurred.

This is a young man whose early feelings of rage at the loss of his mother may have threatened to overwhelm his psyche. He had to get rid of these in the only way he could, by projecting them violently into a recipient that fulfilled his unconscious criteria. Any woman (or man) could be a potential victim of his, if they were experienced by him to ignore him, and to behave as if there was nothing the matter. His female victim, who in reality turned away from facing him and was, by all accounts, happily on her way home, could be said to represent the mother who turned her back on him, but she was also the object of his envy since she was free of the disturbance he was full of that moment. Perceiving the woman to be ignoring him and happily going home, he had to defend against the rage and anxiety that his feelings of motherlessness and homelessness provoked in him but which he felt had been provoked by the object. Instead of feeling at the mercy of a cruel and abandoning object, he attempted to control the object by the attack. One could say that it was not her handbag he was trying to steal but her sense of, in his mind, undeserved well-being.

This offence has profound transferential implications. In the early years of his therapy, one way he tried to defend against the perceived attacks on his psyche was by presenting himself to me as knowing exactly what he needed and demanding this. When he experienced the inevitable frustrations of his unmet demands, or, when he discovered that he was not in control of his object, me, he could become furious. This could be triggered by, for example, me saying that the session had ended. The loss of omnipotently created control of his object led to a fury, in those early years of treatment that had no other way of being experienced other than discharging itself violently. This was indeed one way he had developed to avoid a repeat of any further losses – omnipotently attempting to control those around him. I am referring to when the patient actually required treatment in the intensive care unit of the high security hospital, during which time the therapy was able to proceed in a glass room with two nurses sitting outside, seeing but not hearing.

A similar situation could arise when, occasionally, I was not what and how he wanted me to be. He could either respond with fury, when he would shout angrily at me or walk out before 'losing it'. Alternatively, he experienced being the victim of my psychic assault on his mind.

During these two kinds of moments, Mr. A is highly dangerous. In the first situation, that of losing his omnipotent control of his object, his propensity to act violently towards me or somebody else on the ward is massively increased momentarily, or, at least until that particular state of mind subsides. In the second situation, the risk of dangerousness is greater against himself, when he might deliberately harm himself whilst he feels himself to be my victim. He can be simultaneously identified with both aggressor and victim as well as expertly projecting these into me. The experience of being his therapist is that one could be made to feel very anxious and frightened at those intense moments and it was important to use those feelings constructively to formulate the best interpretation under the difficult circumstances, speaking to the patient informatively about what he was then doing to me, his object.

At other times, this patient has presented himself as innocent and harmless, as a nice young man. At these moments, the patient is sufficiently disturbed to believe his delusion of being a nice young man who is misunderstood. This presentation can be very convincing as well as alluring and professionals, including me, have had to work hard not to be taken in. One way of trying to avoid feeling anxious and frightened whilst being with such a patient is to collude with what Leslie Sohn referred to as their delusion of sanity (Sohn [personal communication, 2010]). This is when serious errors of clinical judgement can be made. To reassure the patient at this moment might well function as a sedative for both patient and therapist, but the 'reassured' states are temporary and can swiftly shift to a more obvious hostile presentation. For example, the patient was telling me about his feelings for a nurse he had developed an eroto-manic attachment to and later in the session, spoke excitedly about another patient who hated her and wanted to kill her. I eventually addressed his feeling like killing her before considering addressing this in the transference to me and he screamed at me in response, 'How can you say that? You treat me as if I was a dangerous person?' Another time, he agitatedly paced around the room, furious about having been secluded after threatening to smash up the ward. He shouted at me 'Don't they know yet that I am not a danger!' At these moments, the patient's awareness of who and how he is, is not available to him. I, in order to retain a useful psychoanalytic stance, have to be prepared to remind him what he definitely does not want reminded of. This interpretation can be experienced as an attempt by me to kill him, albeit psychically, which he needs to defend himself against. Again we have a moment of increased risk of dangerousness when he might get rid of his feelings by acting them out. The next immediate interpretation therefore needs to be to show the patient how, when he is reminded of who and how he is, he feels traumatized by this. The hope is that when this has been repeated in therapy hundreds of times, each time it may become less necessary for this to be a bodily experience of rage and terror by the patient and more able to be experienced in his mind.

This patient remains in treatment and we anticipate that, after another 1–2 years in high security, he should be well enough to manage the transfer to medium security.

### Case 2

Mr. C is a 27-year-old man who was detained in hospital for nine years under a Hospital Order from the court. He was in high security for the first seven years, in medium security for the following two years and was discharged to the community just over one year ago. Mr. C killed his mother and was convicted of manslaughter.

He grew up in a very deprived part of London. He is the eldest of two sons by his teenage mother's relationship that broke down when they were very young and resulted in no further contact.

Mr. C's mother was seriously alcoholic and described in one social worker's report as 'preferring a can of beer to her own children'. She seriously neglected her children, herself and her home. There are descriptions of her repeatedly telling her children they were 'a piece of shit'. For Mr. C to be told this may have led to the belief that his mother could only produce shit and this has had strong implications in the transference, especially early on when I was suspected by the patient of dressing up as a therapist/mother when all I would offer him was 'shit'.

Mr. C truanted frequently, but it was not until the age of nine years that he was referred to professionals because of serious behavioural problems. He then attended a special school for disturbed boys but this school also expelled him. Between 10 and 12 years of age, he ran away from home regularly, lived on the streets, belonging to a gang of older boys who all took drugs and committed burglaries. In other words, this was a boy who had a totally dysfunctional existence with loss of any parental guidance whatsoever.

When he was 12 years old, his mother was asked to bring him to a Family Court. He did apparently feel anxious that he was going to be taken away into care and asked his mother for reassurance. She apparently told him not to worry, she would not let them do this, she would look after him. When it was his mother's turn to speak in court, she began complaining bitterly about how awful he was and how she could not cope with him and asked the court to take him away. This is in fact the moment we think his mother received, unbeknown to him or her, her death sentence.

He was in fact placed in different care homes, all of which he kept running away from. Due to ongoing absconding, he was sent to a long-term children's home far from his London where he stayed for three years. This was the first settled period to date in his life where he thrived, academically and socially.

After turning 16 years, he was promoted to what was called a cluster flat within this children's home, to acknowledge increasing capacity for independence. He was thrilled by this but experienced it as a stressful demand. He dealt with his inability to manage this by burgling another of the cluster flats. He was charged and taken to court. The judge dealt with this unbelievably by forbidding him to return to the home and instead, telling the probation officer to give him a train ticket back to London – that he did not deserve what had been offered to him. He therefore left the children's home with no preparation whatsoever, had no choice but to return to stay at his mother's and within two months, she was dead.

On the day of the killing, he had been drinking heavily with her since early morning. They ran out of alcohol after several hours and she insisted that he go out to buy some more. A row ensued during which time she repeatedly called him a piece of shit. At this moment, (on the background of experiencing the rejection by the children's home) his illusion of shared time with a drinking mate/mother may have shattered when he realised he was only her means of getting alcohol, in other words, merely an object to satisfy her. He told me that he could not tolerate the demands she was making and he 'cracked up' and attacked her. She fell unconscious to the floor and he believed that she was feigning being dead. He proceeded to attack her ferociously in his psychotic state of belief that she was still a danger to his survival, until she was obliterated. He then slept in the same room, woke up the next morning, stepped over her body and went out to the shops, even buying alcohol for her. Later that day he was arrested. He denied having killed his mother and it is likely that he believed this, as he appears to have been in a dissociated state, which enabled him to go to sleep and to get up the next morning as though nothing had happened.

On admission to high secure hospital, Mr. C was noted to be impulsive, abusive, jovial or clowning around and always pushing boundaries. He started to attend some treatment forums and work centres, but this was considered to be compliant behaviour on his part with one objective, to get out. This detachment from any truth about himself and his history was maintained until he started therapy which was his first experience of being with a person who showed consistent interest in him and repeatedly questioned his laughing and joking things off, considering how serious the predicament was for a young man, himself, in this hospital for having killed his mother. Slowly, Mr. C began to take himself more seriously. He gradually discovered that he had a thing called a mind that he could make use of.

Early on, sessions with me began with a chirpy jocular entrance and an attempt to turn me into a social visit and far away from anything serious. If I interpreted his use of jokiness as a defence against seriousness, he could experience this as too demanding. When demands became too much, he had to get rid of these, stop me affecting him, just like he stopped his mother. He would ask me to shut up and eventually, was able to describe the violent fantasies about me that filled his mind at those moments. Here is a session extract from the beginning:

> The patient flew into the room, talking fast with excitement and giggling. 'My case conference went great, all I need is a bit more group work, a bit more talking to you and then I'm out of here' I tried in vain to take up his omnipotent stance where he felt that he could lead the clinical team and me wherever he wanted. 'No' he shouted, 'I just don't care. Yippee, it's great, I don't give a fuck!' He danced around the room singing.

Another feature that came up was his tendency to become high, even without actual drugs available. He would, for example, deprive himself of sleep the nights before his sessions in order to feel high during them. He could not yet trust himself to be sad and needed his manic defence desperately, increasingly so as I interpreted this to him. In the second year he said,

> In fact, I'm not well at all but … I can't say that to them (the team). You know the kind of thoughts I get in my mind. And they are all saying how well I'm doing. I'm just as fucked up now as before, worse in fact because I can see it

His developing sense of curiosity in himself and diminution in his terror of his 'mad' parts were impressive. He gradually became able to experience me, as a good object but not perfect, in other words, not idealised in his previously manic world but not a demonised shit producer either. In a session just before he left high security, he came calmly into the room, sat down and told me that he had moved rooms and had spent all the previous day cleaning out his new thoroughly. It had been absolutely filthy to start off with and was now much cleaner but there was still a bit to go. I nodded with an expression of 'Yes, we know about that'. He smiled a grin indicating he understood. He then told me there had been an incident, which had troubled him. A patient who wanted a chat had come to his door whilst he was cleaning the new room and sat down outside it. The patient had lit a cigarette and Mr. C noticed this, knowing it to be against the rules but said nothing although he felt uncomfortable, as it was right outside his door. Two nurses checking the corridor area noticed the smoking and immediately came to tell the other patient that this was forbidden and took him away. One of those nurses came back to Mr. C and accused him of having offered the light. He felt furious by this accusation and said that in the past, he would have, he knew that, but not anymore. His protests of innocence were ignored. They did not believe him. He then looked up at me questioningly. I said that he was very upset that the nurses, and maybe I, still thought of him as how he used to be and not how he feels himself to be now, much 'cleaner' but still a bit to go.

The continuity in therapy and therapist, given his particular history of inconsistencies, abandonments and losses, was particularly important. This was a young man who had never been able to experience sad feelings but instead, had developed a formidable manic repertoire to defend against these, which had failed him miserably and tragically. Continuity offered him the opportunity to further develop his internal world shifts towards a healthier way of responding to external events particularly those reminiscent of earlier experiences. The move from high security, albeit highly desired by him, (like the promotion to the cluster flat earlier) was complicated by the additional experience of feeling abandoned or even betrayed by high security, like he had been by the residential home and earlier still, by his mother. The difference was that he was able to recognise his states of mind and speak about the feelings engendered this time. Just before leaving high security, he said to me

> You know, I'm so pleased to have made it to this stage and moving on but there is a part of me that would like to simply live in a nice little cottage in the grounds of this hospital. Then I could be sure you and the team had not overestimated me and if things went wrong, I'd still be in the right place.

Simultaneously, the patient had to manage experiencing guilt due to his capacity for remorse and for having got better which led him to feel suicidal periodically.

After one year of me travelling to see him in his new unit, he began to be escorted to the Portman Clinic[1] for sessions. On his first occasion of coming to see me, he said upon entering my consulting room 'Wow, it's great to come and see you, to be here, at last – we MADE it!' a not untypical manic response to feeling anxious. Eventually, he made the journey alone. This 'promotion' led to the first of several minor re-enactments. After this session, instead of travelling straight back to hospital, he deviated to his old home territory, met up with past 'colleagues' who celebrated his visit with alcohol and the offer of 'work'. He then telephoned me in an intoxicated state asking for help. I interpreted this to him in his next session not just as his re-enactment of how he responded to earlier 'promotions' but also as his way of checking to see if he had indeed changed and also seeking reassurance that his old self was alive and kicking. This one incident took several months of sessions to be dissected and understood.

This patient has since been discharged to his own flat, attends evening college, works during the day and travels a long distance every week for his therapy sessions.

## Discussion

The aim of the therapy, as part of the overall treatment, is to attempt to gradually help the patients develop knowledge of themselves, what they have done and what kind of mental life they lived before, including their experiences and responses to traumatic losses, that allowed these awful events. Given their diagnoses of severe personality disorder and therefore damaged mental structure, how can this be achieved using a psychoanalytic approach? I believe it can by offering, over many years, a consistent interpreting stance, provided in a supportive manner. This can only work in the context of support from the clinical team who are regularly informed by the therapist of mental state changes and in the context of the physical security which provides the necessary external boundaries before internal boundaries have formed. With the regular feedback, clinical team members can be alert to the anticipated patient provocations and offer unified therapeutic responses and not unprocessed mixed counter-transferential responses that can otherwise arise (Stasch, 2004)). The communication between therapist and clinical team offers the patient a new model of consistent 'parenting' where the 'parents' communicate thoughtfully about the patient instead of exposing the patient to frightening and perplexing violent actions. The changes that are seen to arise and which I hope to have illustrated clinically are in several areas and I will describe these using the Operationalized Psychodynamic Diagnostics (OPD Task Force, 2001) mental structure model.

The first necessary change in the damaged mental structures, I believe, arises in the area of attachment, or with the capacity to begin introjecting new objects. The chance to relate differently is fostered by offering a stable, balanced person to relate to over a long period of time, in other words, offering object constancy, which the patients have never had. Further changes in other aspects of structural dimensions then have the chance to germinate. Firstly, in self-perception, the patients develop some curiosity about this new situation and after many attempts over years to get the object to respond in the expected way and, in many instances perceiving this to be the case, they become able to take the risk that the object may be different. In the presence of a constant object, albeit one that is still perceived as unpredictable, he or she can gradually develop a capacity for self-reflection. Secondly, after hundreds of occasions identifying the various affects in sessions, patients become aware of these, when they arise (externally or internally provoked) and even eventually to differentiate between them. Simultaneously, the capacity for object perception evolves with concomitant subject–object differentiation, awareness of the affects of the other and thereby, the beginning of capacity for empathy with, much later on in treatment, consequent guilt and remorse, when suicidality can arise. This is when the constellation of post-traumatic stress disorder type symptoms can emerge. With the improved self and object perceptions, attachments gradually become less disordered, communication becomes more reciprocal and the main defence modes, which relate to these other structural dimensions, can mature. Regulation and tolerance of affects can be more internally located and less reliant on external measures. However, it is important to note that, at times of stress, when increased demands are placed on the patients, their mental states can regress and this is when a return to previous functioning, albeit in a modified way, is possible. At these times, patients are prone to minor re-enactments, which cause major anxiety in those looking after them. In other words, the mental structure changes remain fragile and can shift back to being less integrated.

If in infancy, excessive hostility and consequent paranoid anxiety is experienced towards the primary object, the stronger the fixation and the deeper the split between a bad and a highly idealised object. There are consequently transferential complexities that arise from treating people whose primary figures, mother, and symbols of mother, were abandoning, unreliable, replaced and frequently violent objects, leading to the employment of omnipotent defence mechanisms characterised by excessive splitting and projection. In the transference, right from the start, the patient's fixation at paranoid levels of development and their defenses have to be repeatedly analysed in order to eventually mobilise the patient's capacity for experiencing love, depression and guilt.

The patients presented are both diagnosed as suffering from personality disorders, Mr. A, antisocial and narcissistic, Mr. C, antisocial (American Psychiatric Association (APA), 2013; National Institute for Health & Clinical Excellence, 2009). Both became unwell during their adolescence and I believe that these were their second breakdowns, the first having also occurred unnoticed when they were infants or small children and which led to the disordered personality development. The presenting symptoms, consistent with diagnoses of personality disorder, are also consistent with those of a prodromal phase of a psychotic illness, the psychosis becoming manifest at the moment of the killing. The evidence for this is available in the histories. In the months leading up to the killings, these patients became periodically withdrawn, egocentric and grandiose, similar to those young people harbouring a schizophrenic illness. Mr. A came close to killing women on several occasions beforehand and managed to retreat from doing so by still having a sane part of his ego which could overcome the demands to kill coming from the psychotic and mad part of his superego. When he killed the woman, this is the moment that his psychotic illness triumphed over the personality disorder, which was no longer able to defend him against the propensity for enormous splitting and projection and led to a spillage out of the mind into action. Mr. C tried to reason with his drunk mother but, when she persisted in assaulting his illusion that he was with a mother, his personality disorder that had defended him by modifying the degree of splitting and projection, weakened by intoxication, caved in to the demands of a psychotic part of his mind which was deluded that self-preservative violence was necessary in order to survive psychically.

To return to diagnostic clarification, in my view, it is more helpful for us to consider these patients as suffering from a single entity, where at times, the psychotic symptoms are more manifest and at other times, the personality disorder symptoms more so (Hale & Dhar, 2008). This could improve the tendency to split treatments and perpetuate a split in the patients' minds. In other words, I am suggesting that the diagnoses of certain Personality Disorders are synonymous with an earlier missed diagnosis of a prodromal psychotic illness, patients' mental states subsequently vacillating between showing symptoms of psychoses or symptoms of personality disorders.

After several years of treatment, symptoms reminiscent of post-traumatic stress disorder can arise and the evidence for these is: the emergence of flashbacks, nightmares, preoccupation with the awful events that happened to them growing up and those that they later caused, states of mind alternating between being depressed or being manically freed from this and, eventually, a capacity to experience guilt. Due to the structural changes that arise, the experience of remorse can arise and is often accompanied by a complex mixture of depressed and angry feelings with a psychical longing to return to a state of oblivion (OPD Task Force, 2008). Mr. C once said

> It's much worse for me now Doctor, all this thinking and analysing, but I could never go back to how I was before you helped me train the muscles of my mind, even though I'd like to sometimes. Before, if I didn't like something, I'd smash it to pieces. Now, if I don't like something, I start thinking, now, why don't I like that? Oh, it's for this or that reason and so on. By the time I've worked it all out, I don't even feel like smashing it up any more.

To conclude, the process of treatment appears to require a complicated and lengthy transition period from the patient knowing very little about himself, to developing awareness and dealing with the profoundly traumatic effects of this, where thoughts and feelings about what happened and their predicament in relation to this could be experienced in mind without the need to get rid of these in the familiar ways of acting them out violently. With consistency over a long period of time, it is possible for these patients to make tentative shifts towards the 'depressive position' and this is something that needs to be worked through over and over until the negative therapeutic responses, triggered by the positive shifts, or, provoked by 'getting better', lessen in severity and frequency. Long-term continuity of treatment throughout the patient's moves through different levels of security is necessary to enable this to arise. It is a lot to ask of people who suffer the triple traumas described earlier, as well as being a challenge to those treating them. The chance to develop a mind and life which is reliably different can only be realised within the necessary physical security to start off, the mutual commitment of patient and therapist, collaboration with the clinical team and regular supervisions, with reflective practice for all concerned with these patients (Fallon, Bluegrass, Edwards, & Daniels, 1999).

## Disclosure statement

No potential conflict of interest was reported by the author.

## Note

1. The Portman Clinic is a National Health Service outpatient clinic in London, UK, that provides psychoanalytically informed treatments for violent, delinquent and perverse patients.

## References

American Psychiatric Association (APA). (2013). *Diagnostic and statistical manual of mental disorders* (5th ed.). Washington, DC: Author.

Fallon, P., Bluegrass, R., Edwards, B., & Daniels, G. (1999). *The report of the Committee of Inquiry into the Personality Disorder Unit, Ashworth Special Hospital (Cm 4194-II)*. London: The Stationery Office.

Hale, R., & Dhar, R. (2008). Flying a kite – Observations on dual (and triple) diagnosis. *Criminal Behaviour and Mental Health, 18*, 145–152.

Klein, M. (1935). A contribution to the psychogenesis of manic depressive states. In M. Klein (Ed.), *Love, Guilt, Reparation and Other Works 1921–1945* (pp. 262–289). London: Hogarth.

Klein, M. (1946). Notes on some schizoid mechanisms. In M. Klein (Ed.), *Envy and Gratitude and Other Works* (pp. 1–24). London: Hogarth, 1975.

National Institute for Health and Clinical Excellence. (2009). *NICE clinical guideline 77.* Anti-Social Personality Disorder Full Guideline. NICE: London.

OPD Task Force. (2001). *Operationalized psychodynamic diagnostics foundations and manual*. Göttingen: Hogrefe & Huber,

OPD Task Force. (2008). *Operationalized psychodynamic diagnosis OPD-2 manual of DIAGNOSIS and treatment planning*. Seattle, WA: Hegrefe & Huber.

Sohn, L. (1997). Unprovoked assaults in reason and passion. (D. Bell, Editor). London: Karnac Books

Stasch, M. (2004). *Interpersonal tuning in inpatient psychotherapy. A clinical approach based on the Operationalized Psychodynamic Diagnostics (OPD)*. Paper presented at the 34th annual meeting of the Society for Psychotherapy Research, Weimar.

Warren, F. (2003) Review of treatments for severe personality disorder. Home Office Online Report. London: Research Development and Statistics Directorate, Home Office.

# In praise of Dr Leslie Sohn 1919–2013

Dr Leslie Sohn, a world expert on the psychotic mind, an NHS psychiatrist for 62 years, a psychoanalyst (training adult and child analyst), a collector of Chinese antiquities and a lover of flowers, a lifelong supporter of Manchester United FC, a family man, died on 18 March 2013 aged 93 years. Dr Sohn spent his incredibly long working life dedicated to the plight of patients in forensic psychiatry systems and teaching and supervising professionals from the different disciplines involved in their care.

Leslie Sohn was born in Cape Town, 1919, the youngest of three children, having two sisters several years older. He attended the local public day school and then read medicine at the University of Cape Town. His attachment to the psychiatric department of the university hospital produced clear signs of a profound interest in this field. He completed his House Officer posts in Durban and waited for the war to end before coming to England for postgraduate training in psychiatry.

Dr Sohn was delighted to be appointed Senior House Physician in 1947 to Aubrey Lewis at the Maudsley Hospital. In 1948, with the forming of the National Health Service, his attachment became one of Psychiatric Registrar and then, Senior Registrar. The word 'psychoanalysis' had not yet entered his vocabulary. Whilst working at the Maudsley Hospital, he was fortunate to work clinically for Clifford Scott and William Gillespie who inspired his psychoanalytic interest. He was encouraged to apply to the Institute of Psychoanalysis, was accepted and supervised by Marion Milner and Hannah Segal, qualifying in 1952. Two of his peers during the training were Sidney Klein and Isabelle Menzies-Lyth with whom he maintained a friendship over several decades. They continued to meet regularly at postgraduate seminars, including over a period of 12 years at the Rosenfeld seminar, where Sohn and Klein presented. A similar pattern took place at the Segal postgraduate seminar over many years.

Throughout this time, Dr Sohn continued working at the Maudsley Hospital and, post-qualification as a psychoanalyst, began to develop his private practice. He also completed the Child Psychoanalytic training.

Dr Sohn's loyalty and compassion for disturbed and disturbing patients, and in particular his respect for the nurses caring for them, were truly astonishing. His relationships with certain colleagues were at times more tricky but always honest. His psychoanalytic insights, always invaluable, were offered constantly in a generous way although he occasionally expressed his dismay that no one else's mind could spark in the same way or at the same speed. He was known for his rather sophisticated humour as well as his poetic way of describing the world and his incredible capacity for lateral thinking. In the sense that Richard Lucas, also taught by Dr Sohn, wrote about in his book, *The Psychotic Wavelength* (Lucas, 2009), no one was more able to tune into this wavelength than Dr Sohn, meaning he had an understanding of patients that no one else could quite get. Furthermore, he never forgot the histories of any of the hundreds of patients that were presented to him over the decades. If he was presented with a particularly disturbing or puzzling case by a trainee, at the next meeting, the trainee would discover that Dr Sohn had spent the weekend walks thinking about the case and have a succinct understanding of what had previously been baffling. He never ceased to think and was a great supporter of introducing patients to the fact they had a mind, albeit a hurt and damaged one, and one that they could use differently. He applied the same approach to professionals, constantly introducing supervisees to tune into the less conscious aspects of patients' presentations, in order to deepen their understanding of the patients' minds and consequent behaviours.

Dr Sohn maintained his position as Consultant Psychiatrist at the Maudsley Hospital from 1952 until 1995. He was then appointed as Consultant Psychiatrist at Broadmoor High Security Hospital, where he worked until 2010, aged 90 years. This means that Dr Sohn was employed in the NHS for a period of 62 years seamlessly (1948–2010). During this time, Dr Sohn assessed and treated hundreds of patients and supervised and inspired hundreds of juniors, from medical and other disciplines, excelling as a clinician and teacher. In particular, his attachment to the Medium Secure Unit at the Bethlem Royal Hospital (Dennis Hill Unit) revolutionized the way of thinking about and understanding violent behaviour in mentally disordered offenders and in particular, those suffering from psychotic illnesses. He especially enjoyed working alongside his colleagues in forensic psychiatry, Dr James Mc Keith, Professor John Gunn and Professor Pamela Taylor. His paper 'Unprovoked assaults' (Sohn, 1995) was particularly influential in providing a way of understanding the apparently inexplicable, sudden and often bizarre, violent offences carried out by mentally ill patients, indicating that there was indeed a provocation, albeit a complex psychical one arising from traumatic historical events, where the victim of the assault becomes a suitable external recipient for the extreme projections that are enacted bodily through the violent act.

Another major contribution was his paper 'Narcissistic organisation, projective identification, and the formation of the identificate' (Sohn, 1985), where he was the first to take further what happens within narcissistic organizations in psychotic cases. To quote him

> an identification via projective identification has taken place, which heightens omnipotence, to allow what has been termed the identificate to believe that it has become the desired object – and thereby that within this spuriously organized ego-structure exist the characteristics and functions of the object or part-object that has been taken over.... The functions of these 'successful defense' manoeuvres are to obviate any feelings or awareness of envy... secondly, they nullify any awareness of dependence... or need or of illness...and thirdly they maintain the narcissistic organization by producing a successful identificate. (Sohn, 1985, p. 213)

This groundbreaking theoretical understanding led on to another major contribution to the work with psychiatry and that is, to beware of the patients' presenting as 'sane', their illness being consequently overlooked or underestimated and hence, left untreated.

He was a pioneer in developing a highly sophisticated form of reflective practice for forensic mental health clinicians at all levels of seniority, now Department of Health guidance for all forensic psychiatry settings (Department of Health Secure Services Policy Team, 2010). He published several papers in the International Journal of Psychoanalysis. One of his most interesting and useful theoretical developments has been that of considering a mad part of the psychotic patient's superego envying what goes on between patient and analyst and repeatedly attempting to 'assault' the therapeutic process. His repeated reminders to clinicians working in forensic psychiatry settings of the constant need to watch out for 'collusions with delusions of sanity' have had a major impact on the training of clinicians from different disciplines as well as ameliorating the care provided to patients in these settings, where there is a strong tendency for such collusions to arise. This has also had repercussions in risk assessment and management of patients who have been violent.

Right up until his death, Dr Sohn continued working in private practice and providing supervision for clinicians working in the NHS and in private practice. In June 2000, he and Dr Minne set up a monthly Forensic Psychoanalysis seminar at the Institute of Psychoanalysis for interested clinicians, attending in person or via teleconferencing from abroad. This continues as the monthly Sohn Seminar, attended by professionals from seven different countries – and expanding. A collection of his papers, many unpublished as he prioritized seeing patients and trainees, is being prepared for publication.

Dr Sohn had four children with his beloved Myra, who died in 1995. If he was not out adding to his collection of Chinese antiquities, or watching Manchester United FC, he spent his free time with his four children, Nicola, Tracey, Philippa and Hughie, nine grandchildren and five great grand children. He was a dedicated family man as well as a most generous extraordinary teacher. Conferences abroad with him were opportunities to get to know other sides of him, like his wicked sense of humour, his shopping sprees, his enjoyment of social outings and entertaining people with a variety of stories, each one more astounding than the next! He died somewhat unexpectedly and peacefully on 18 March 2013, surrounded by his close family. It is my privilege to have known him, learnt so much from him over 23 precious years, and my sadness to experience the loss of an extraordinary man.

## References

Department of Health Secure Services Policy Team (2010). *See, Think, Act.* London: Department of Health.

Lucas, R. (2009). *The psychotic wavelength, a psychoanalytic perspective for psychiatry.* (New Library of Psychoanalysis). London: Routledge.

Sohn, L. (1985). Narcissistic organization, projective identification, and the formation of the identificate. *International Journal of Psychoanalysis, 66*, 201–213.

Sohn, L. (1995). Unprovoked assaults - making sense of apparently random violence. *International Journal of Psychoanalysis, 78*, 565–575.

Carine Minne

# A fertile matrix: the birth of the Forensic Psychotherapy Society

Gabriel Kirtchuk[a], John Gordon[a], Ronald Doctor[b] and Richard Ingram[c]

[a]*Forensic Psychotherapy Department, West London Mental Health NHS Trust, London, UK;* [b]*Psychotherapy Service, West London Mental Health NHS Trust, West Middlesex Hospital, Isleworth, UK;* [c]*Centre for Psychotherapy, Belfast Trust, Belfast, UK*

This paper traces some aspects of the fertile matrix within which, over many years, the application of a psychoanalytic perspective to clinical work with the most severely mentally ill, difficult and at times frightening patients in secure and community settings has evolved and now led to the recent inauguration of the Forensic Psychotherapy Society (FPS), a new Member Institution of the British Psychoanalytic Council. The Society provides both a framework for a national, multidisciplinary professional training in psychodynamic forensic psychotherapy and the potential launching pad for an active post-qualification organisation supporting CPD and all other forms of professional development. The particular contributions to the birth of the FPS of the Forensic Psychotherapy Department at West London Mental Health NHS Trust, partly because we know it best but also because it is part of the largest forensic psychiatric service in the United Kingdom, are described.

Forensic Psychotherapy is the application of a psychoanalytic perspective to clinical work with the most severely ill, difficult and at times frightening patients in secure and community settings. The matrix within which it has developed contains deep and wide historical roots. Mervyn Glasser, Adam Limentani, Robert Hale, Donald Campbell and Estela Welldon at the Portman Clinic, among many others working independently such as Arthur Hyatt-Williams and Patrick Gallwey, have made major contributions. Murray Cox and Leslie Sohn at Broadmoor Hospital, along with their colleagues, expanded understanding of complex forensic psychopathology in the high security hospital. The International Association of Forensic Psychotherapy, spearheaded by Estela Welldon, enabled larger gatherings of professionals in the field to present their clinical work and extend their skills. The purpose of this paper is to indicate some other current and significant components of this fertile matrix and to describe how the resulting training structures and opportunities for clinicians working in this complex area were transformed to create the Forensic Psychotherapy Society (FPS), a new Member Institution of the British Psychoanalytic Council (BPC).

**Origins of a National Forensic Psychotherapy Training structure**

In 1997 an inquiry into the Personality Disorder Unit (PDU) at Ashworth Special Hospital (The Fallon Inquiry) was commissioned following allegations by a patient of serious and pervasive boundary violations. These alleged breaches of care and security included 'the misuse of drugs and alcohol, financial irregularities, possible paedophile activity and the availability of pornographic material on the Unit' (Report of the Committee of Inquiry, 1999). The allegations were found 'to be largely accurate. Pornography was widely available on the ward; patients were running their own businesses; hospital policies were ignored; and security was grossly inadequate' (Ibid.). Scathingly, the Inquiry concluded that the PDU '... was a deeply flawed creation. A number of highly serious reports have demonstrated Ashworth Hospital's failure to care for and manage a large group of severely personality disordered patients' (Ibid.). Finally – and crucially for the training developments traced in this account – the Committee members emphasised deficits in the capacity to formulate and think about (in effect, to contain) the emotional turbulence of contact with severe personality disorder: 'The focus of clinical discussion and decision-making was predominantly on social behaviour and administrative and risk issues, rather than on seeking a psychological understanding of the patient' (Ibid.).

In response to this emergency and these clinical concerns, Robert Hale from the Portman Clinic was influential in negotiating with the Department of Health to establish nine 5-year dual training posts in Forensic Psychotherapy where doctors in higher psychiatric training could train in both psychoanalytic psychotherapy and forensic psychiatry. Subsequently, West London Mental Health NHS Trust joined the Portman Clinic to add a further two posts.

The rationale was that doctors with such a dual training would be much better equipped to enhance multidisciplinary teams' awareness of the often unconscious dynamics arising from patients' early experiences and to consider the reverberating emotional impacts which determined relationships between patients and professionals on the wards and in other mental health settings. Accordingly, the 'psychological understanding of the patient' stressed in the Fallon Report (Fallon, Bluglass, Edwards, & Daniels, 1999) could be addressed. However, such a small number of isolated psychodynamically informed clinicians spread across the United Kingdom required the development of a peer group to consolidate their identity in this new specialty as well as to provide continuing training.

Consequently, with the support of the Department of Health (particularly that of Eddie Kane) and of the Royal College of Psychiatrists, the National Strategy for Forensic Training and Education, chaired by Gill McGauley with Gabriel Kirtchuk as Lead Clinician, was formed to support the dual trainees and to anticipate and meet subsequent training requirements. This development was actively augmented by the participation of several prominent Forensic Psychiatrists: Robert Dolan, Pamela Taylor, Janet Parrott and David Reiss, among others. In this context and with the support of Chris Mace, then Chair of the Psychotherapy Faculty of the Royal College of Psychiatry, a Forensic Psychotherapy Special Interest Group was established at the College initially under the chairmanship of Carine Minne.

In retrospect, the next phase was obvious: the relatively small number of medical trainees would never expand to the point of creating a critical mass of psychodynamically skilled professionals who could have a decisive impact within forensic services. Therefore, a proposal to develop a pilot project for a multidisciplinary training leading to a Forensic Practitioner-level qualification was considered by the National Strategy for Forensic Training and Education. The Forensic Psychotherapy Department at West London Mental Health NHS Trust was well placed to take on this project due to several circumstances. First, it was the only Forensic Psychotherapy Department within a Medium Secure Unit with an expanded remit in training and education. Second, it operated within a trust that has the largest and most comprehensive forensic psychiatric services in the country. Finally, it inherited a prolonged experience of using basic psychoanalytic concepts to train a wide range of multidisciplinary professionals within this rich clinical context. This strand of the matrix, long pre-dating the Ashworth Inquiry with which our story began, will now be described.

## The MSc

The two-year MSc in Psychotherapeutic Approaches in Mental Health is a collaboration between the Forensic Psychotherapy Training Department at West London Mental Health NHS Trust and New Buckinghamshire University. This training for multidisciplinary professionals working in general and forensic psychiatric hospitals, community mental health and associated services (social services, general practice, probation) applies a psychoanalytic perspective to understand the individual, group and organisational dynamics which permeate their work.

The current MSc is the culmination of a long development which originated in Bob Hinshelwood's Psychotherapy Department at St Bernard's Hospital at WLMH NHS Trust. In the late 1980s, Bob, David Riley and John Gordon organised a training at the request of the on-site School of Nursing which offered nurses an opportunity to experience and learn about group dynamics and group psychotherapy.

Subsequently, Gabriel Kirtchuk joined the Psychotherapy Department and devised a Training in Psychodynamic Assessment to which Bob Hinshelwood, David Riley and John Gordon also contributed. A major elaboration of these early ventures then took shape in order to recognise the increasing importance of more advanced academic qualifications for nurses.

Gabriel Kirtchuk, John Gordon and Beatrice Stevens negotiated with Ellen Noonan, Head of the Counselling Section at Birkbeck College, University of London, to establish a Certificate/Diploma in Work with the Mentally Ill in Hospital and Community.

Although not involved directly in the planning, Bob Hinshelwood (soon to be the first External Examiner for the West London/Birkbeck Certificate/Diploma) remained in touch with us throughout. In a letter to Gabriel on 20 June 1996, he conveyed congratulations and his always thought-provoking reflections on the new venture:

> I want to raise one rather basic issue, which might affect the kind of teaching on the course, and the kind of students who come on it. As a course primarily for nurses, it seems to me that there might be some space on the course for an 'integrative' kind of activity to consider the nurses' medical model approach in relation to the 'talking cure' type of approach which the course represents. Working with mentally ill patients is quite a serious and arduous project, and the limits of counseling are obvious. It seems to me that the danger is that nurses can use their new understanding to become, as it were, roving interpreters. As we know, the verbal containing has to take place in a very specific setting. To some extent the question of using psychoanalytically based insights outside the analytic consulting room is a research activity ... It seems to me the course might reflect the fundamental difference of approach ... and give space for students (and staff) to consider the problems, conflicts and paradoxes that arise.

We wrestled with this and many other dilemmas involved in teaching applied psychodynamics over the next 13 years, during which time we were joined by Maya Jarrett from Birkbeck and subsequently by the late Carola Gross from Bob's former Psychotherapy Department who took over teaching basic psychoanalytic concepts when Beatrice Stevens retired. The course structure remained constant: an academic seminar in which papers from the core psychoanalytic, group and systems theory literature were presented and discussed; an application group in which students presented process accounts of clinical material from work with individual patients and observations of/work in groups, to which the academic concepts and models would be applied; an Experiential Group; and a group relations event held at Birkbeck College.

At the end of his term, Bob Hinshelwood was succeeded as External Examiner by Marco Chiesa and then Kingsley Norton. Gill McGauley is the current External Examiner. Over 150 students, mainly nurses but also occupational therapists, social workers, 'creative' (arts, music and drama) therapists and a few doctors completed this Certificate/Diploma. Their feedback was always illuminating as the following examples reveal. A CPN in the EMI team wrote: 'It gave me a lot of insight into working with the anxieties about growing old experienced by my patients and helped me to contain them.' A Care Manager at a Community Mental Health Centre emphasised another aspect:

> The course helped me to understand the group dynamics taking place in my resource centre and to reflect more on the personal impact of the work on myself. It's given me an insight into previously confusing emotional interactions with patients. It's really got me thinking.

A GP commented:

> I have learned a more meaningful appreciation of human relationships after attending this course and have developed a more searching attitude whilst solving problems that exist in my clinical practice. The course has given me the confidence to enter into my patients' inner worlds to identify emotional reasons for presenting complaints and symptoms.

Finally, a Senior Nurse at a Community Mental Health Resource Centre observed:

> Initially it was daunting and I felt, 'What is this about?', but as the course went on I began to understand the relevance not only to my work but to my life. Professionally, it's helped to understand personality disordered patients and especially how I am affected by them.

The course staff are aware that some students, as Bob Hinshelwood mentioned, can initially behave like over enthusiastic converts to the new cause, not only acting as though they are Psychotherapists but also interpreting the behaviour of their colleagues. These tendencies are carefully monitored, particularly in the Application Groups where students present verbatim clinical material.

Towards the end of what came to be called the 'Birkbeck Course' period, once again developments in nursing education prompted a major change in our thinking about the course. Over 50% of applicants now already had BSc degrees. Nursing training had itself moved off-site and was based at Buckinghamshire New University which, because of its educational contract with the Trust, presented itself as a potential new partner. Negotiations with several members of the University administration eventuated in the establishment of the current MSc, which was strongly encouraged and supported by Nick Broughton, Medical Director of West London Mental Health NHS Trust and Michael Maier, Head of the School of Psychiatry, London Deanery.

The first student cohort started in September 2010. Core teaching staff include Ronald Doctor, John Gordon, Gabriel Kirtchuk, Maggie McAlister and Beate Schumacher. A 'satellite' development of the MSc in Northern Ireland, led by Richard Ingram and others, will be described below.

## The curriculum

The current MSc is a two-year course composed of four modules: Psychotherapeutic Approaches to Working with Individuals; Psychotherapeutic Approaches to Working with Groups and Organisations; Interpersonal Dynamic Consultation; and Dissertation. The first three modules explicitly envisage the application of psychoanalytic thinking (including attachment and mentalisation-based theories) to three key areas with which students, as professional clinicians, are concerned:

work with individuals and sometimes with patient groups but always within a group and an institutional dynamic context which both fundamentally shape all interventions within the system.

Module three, the Interpersonal Dynamic Consultation, teaches students a manualised (Reiss & Kirtchuk, 2009: Reiss and Kirtchuk, n.d. Kirtchuk, Gordon, McAlister, & Reiss, 2013) protocol for carrying out consultations to ward and community teams. Individual patients referred for this consultation will usually be causing problems for the multidisciplinary professionals involved in their containment, treatment and care. The aim of the consultation is to elicit from staff most involved with the patient the core interpersonal patterns regularly evoked in interactions between the patient and his/her significant others, including the staff, in the present and the past. This is accomplished through applying a structured list of descriptions of how (1) the patient repeatedly perceives others; (2) how the patient in response repeatedly experiences him/herself; (3) how others repeatedly perceive the patient; and (4) how others in response characteristically experience themselves. These four perspectives basically describe any interpersonal interaction, and the descriptors used are jargon-free.

However, it is clear that from the psychodynamic orientation of the MSc we are aiming to provide students with a method of discovering the transference–countertransference scenarios which are unconsciously enacted and reenacted by the patient and others. These scenarios are often profoundly maladaptive, however entrenched their defensive functions, and they can evoke equally maladaptive, even destructive, automatic reactions from staff. Alerting staff to their potential for such reactions by tracing how their patients' impacts are affecting them is a fundamental part of applied psychodynamics. Students are expected to carry out two consultations and to develop increasingly complex formulations of the material to feedback to their teams.

The fourth, Dissertation, module surveys quantitative and qualitative research methods and attempts to introduce psychodynamic aspects of qualitative research such as that exemplified in the work of Wendy Hollway (2001). Qualitative approaches have so far been the predominant choice of students who tend to focus their research on phenomenological accounts of aspects of their work by means of focus groups and semi-structured interviews with mental health staff in their hospital or community settings. This type of research project usually requires only Audit Committee approval and so avoids long delays associated with the Ethics Committee process. Unfortunately, this means that patient-based research is not possible within the short time span of the training, but there have been very interesting studies of, for example, ward reflective practice groups, clinical supervision and CPN involvement with patients' benefit claims. In particular, a service evaluation of Reflective Practice based on focus group interviews with multidisciplinary team members found significant negative elements in their experiences of group facilitators: prolonged silences: not being explicit about the task; and in some cases using too much jargon in their interventions. On the other hand, positive feedback included the opportunity to discuss difficult feelings; the experience of being listened to and the creation of a more coherent staff approach to patients. The findings of this dissertation where presented at trust level and integrated into Clinical Governance recommendations for Reflective Practice.

### The course day

As mentioned above, each teaching day of the MSc is divided into three elements. First students attend an academic seminar in which assigned papers are discussed with a member of the teaching staff. In Module 1, Psychotherapeutic Approaches to Working with Individuals, these papers from the psychoanalytic literature cover early emotional development and the unconscious mind structured by deficit/conflict, internal working models and internalised self-affect–object relationships, the paranoid–schizoid and depressive positions, splitting and projective identification, transference and countertransference and the team as container.

In Module 2, Psychotherapeutic Approaches to Working with Groups and Organisations, papers from the wider literature on group dynamics as well as on group therapy are covered. There is a particular focus on projective processes in groups, a theme which is extended when the Tavistock/Group Relations systemic framework for understanding organisations is introduced. Bion's *Experiences In Groups* is read closely.

In Module 3, papers from the literature on the origins of the Interpersonal Dynamic Consultation, internalised self-object relations in personality disorders, perversions and other pathologies, and psychodynamic formulation are discussed. The format is for a student to present a summary of each paper which acts as the launching pad for discussion. Modules 3 and 4 run concurrently throughout the second year, and there are academic seminars on research methodology which may also be further discussed in the Application Groups.

The second element of the day is the Application Group. This is a form of work study group made up of 5–8 students who in turn present an interaction/session with an individual patient (Module 1), an observation of a group interaction (Module 2) or the results of an ID consultation (Module 3). Every student will have an opportunity to present at least twice during each 15-week module. The task of the group is to discuss the presented process account by applying the theories and concepts from the academic seminars to the clinical material. Gradually students become more able to make use of the psychodynamic perspective and to integrate it with the types of treatment interventions inherent in their specific professional roles.

The final element of the day is the Experiential Group. The task of the group is for students to learn about their responses to being a member of a group – how group membership affects the ways in which individuals feel, think and behave – by getting in touch with and sharing their experiences of the group in the here and now. Wider concerns as members of the course also inevitably emerge in the group meetings.

This combination of academic, clinical and experiential learning is fundamental to the MSc and links it securely to students' professional roles and responsibilities. Consequently, the MSc is viewed as extremely valuable by Trust managers who know from experience how graduates contribute to their ward and community settings as well as to the work of their colleagues.

## The MSc lifts off to Northern Ireland

The MSc in Psychotherapeutic Approaches 'satellite' training in Northern Ireland has been established now for four years and represents a feasible and effective example of how to develop the opportunity for a multi-professional Forensic Psychotherapy Training in a periphery of the United Kingdom in which there is a relatively modest provision of psychoanalytically trained clinicians.

Approximately seven years ago Richard Ingram, along with interested psychiatry trainees, began travelling on a monthly basis from Belfast to Gabriel Kirtchuk's Forensic Psychotherapy Training Department at West London Mental Health NHS Trust to train in the Interpersonal Dynamics Consultation model which had been established there. This association developed further into a weekly teleconferenced workshop in which consultations conducted in London, Belfast and other interested services in the United Kingdom were discussed and formatted in accordance with the Interpersonal Dynamics Consultation model.

Through this contact, psychiatry trainees and other multi-professional staff in Northern Ireland expressed a keen interest in enrolling in the MSc held in London. Funding was found for three candidates who flew over on a rather arduous weekly basis to attend the first year of the course in London. However, through the skills acquired by psychoanalytically trained staff in Belfast in the Interpersonal Dynamics Consultation model at the weekly workshop, it was decided to run the second year of the course (in which this model is taught) for the Belfast MSc candidates in their home city.

With a small core team of four staff at the Department of Psychotherapy in the Belfast Health and Social Care Trust (Derya Courtney, Chris Fry, Richard Ingram and Deirdre Meehan) the 'satellite' MSc was then established with the help of West London Mental Health NHS Trust and Buckinghamshire New University and now runs with a new intake every two years of ten candidates. Core funding for places was obtained from both the Northern Ireland Department of Health and the local Health and Social Care Board to facilitate applications from multi-professional disciplines working throughout mental health services in Northern Ireland. The funding, which was key to developing and sustaining the training, was obtained in the teeth of some of the worst funding conditions in the NHS. This was largely as a result of how persuasive the model of training was in terms of developing the innate skills and psychological intelligence available in multi-disciplinary teams to maximise the effectiveness of teamwork in managing severely disturbed patients. It was therefore regarded as an investment in education and training which would be significantly cost effective in the medium to long term.

It is to be hoped that other regions of the United Kingdom may follow in the manner of this successful collaboration, one in which both centres and peripheries can engage in a mutually rewarding experience of high-quality service development. The publication of the Interpersonal Dynamics Manual and the accessibility of the weekly workshop will now clearly enhance and facilitate potential engagement in this process for other interested regional services. In addition, as will be described shortly, the MSc is now also the initial stage in an escalator model of training for MSc graduates who wish to work towards accreditation as a Forensic Psychotherapist. This higher level of clinical training is also being designed to be accessible to regions and will therefore also be developed in Northern Ireland as a key element in a strategy to develop and more securely establish Forensic Psychotherapy as a discipline in this part of the United Kingdom.

## Integration of medical training in psychotherapy and the MSc

The West London Higher Training in Psychotherapy is a long-established three-year psychotherapy training for ST4–6 doctors in psychoanalytical psychotherapy. (However, the scheme has recently adopted a dual training in Psychotherapy and General Psychiatry as a standard. Therefore, they are ST4–8). There are four posts based in the four West London Mental Health NHS Hospitals – Charing Cross, Ealing, West Middlesex and the Cassel – with one trainee also working part-time at Parkside Clinic. In addition, there are two ST4–8 doctors in Forensic Psychotherapy in conjunction with the Portman Clinic. Medical Directors and Consultants at the Cassel in particular have over many decades made profound contributions to the training of medical psychotherapists. This training, as opposed to most psychotherapy trainings, specifically prepares doctors for working in the NHS with an emphasis on complex and difficult personality disordered patients as well as those with severe and enduring mental illness. Recent Training Programme Directors include Drs David Bell, Gabriel Kirtchuk and Ronald Doctor. Many Psychoanalysts/Consultant Psychotherapists working within the NHS have participated as trainers: Drs Bob Hinshelwood, Roger Kennedy, Kevin Healy, Kami Ghaffari, Bernard Roberts, Marco Chiesa, Brian Martindale, Joan Schachter, Sue Mizan, Kingsley Norton, Wilhelm Skogstadt, Kate Pugh and Anis Janmohamed.

Under Gabriel Kirtchuk and Ronald Doctor, the BPC was approached to try to form an alliance between the NHS West London Training and the external BPC trainings to enable the trainee doctors to attain BPC accreditation on the basis of an academic programme which would satisfy both the BPC and the NHS training criteria. After considerable negotiation, it was decided to form a link with the Lincoln Centre to offer the trainees a first year in the intensive psychoanalytic psychotherapy training: infant observation, academic programme on Freud, Klein and Winnicott and a group clinical seminar on their work in the NHS. This could then be followed by interview to proceed for the full training in intensive psychoanalytic psychotherapy through the Lincoln Centre where one of the two patients seen in psychoanalytical psychotherapy would be an NHS patient seen in the trainee's NHS setting. This approach was highly valued by both the Lincoln Centre and the West London Higher Training in Psychotherapy.

Subsequently, with the development of the new arrangement for all Psychotherapy Training Schemes in London to be placed under a Lead Provider, namely UCL Partnership, the importance of an MSc-level academic component was increasingly emphasised. Accordingly, whilst trainees could continue with the Lincoln Training, now part of the British Psychoanalytic Foundation (BPF), the MSc was incorporated as a core training for doctors in applied psychodynamics. The number of doctors on the MSc immediately increased to 25% or higher, transforming the student cohort – and especially the Experiential Group – into a more multidisciplinary arena with dynamics mirroring students' work environments.

The ST4–6 trainees in The West London Higher Training in Psychotherapy now have a very intensive training in psychoanalytical psychotherapy in the NHS with a joint NHS/external BPC training with the BPF. This innovative, predominantly NHS-based MSc in Psychotherapeutic Approaches to Working with Individuals, Groups and Organisations prepares them for the clinical realities of a career in the NHS.

## Links to the IGA, the BPC and Post-MSc qualification

From the inception it was envisaged that the MSc would develop links to psychotherapy training organisations beyond West London Mental Health NHS Trust and Buckinghamshire New University. Negotiations with the Institute of Group Analysis successfully established the first year of the training, based on the Module 2 focus on group dynamics and particularly on the Experiential Group, as an Introductory (now Foundation) Course equivalent. This enables MSc students who successfully pass Year 1 to apply for full training at the IGA. Further links were made with the BPC which registers graduates of the MSc (who commit themselves to CPD requirements) as Psychodynamic Practitioners/Forensic or General.

A more ambitious proposal builds on all these previous steps and is based on the MSc (or equivalent) as a prerequisite for further training as a multidisciplinary Forensic and/or Generic Psychotherapist as an additional and integrated part of trainees' core clinical profession. The purpose of this training is to increase the number of psychodynamically qualified professionals beyond the current number in order to have a greater impact on increasing demands for talking therapies. Accordingly, we proposed a multi-professional career structure compatible with

CPD requirements which encompasses an escalator model of training with valid and registrable stages of experience. There are two stages.

Stage one is the MSc in Psychotherapeutic Approaches in Mental Health (or equivalent) which leads to a qualification as a Psychodynamic Practitioner/Forensic or General (approved already by BPC). Following the MSc these trainees continue within their normal work setting to practice under supervision. In order to increase the psychodynamic orientation of their work, they would be expected to take on specific roles, for example, as co-facilitators of the ward-based Community Meeting, Reflective Practice and Interpersonal Dynamics Consultations and to act as supervisors to more junior staff, helping them to understand the dynamics of engagement, relational security and boundaries from a dynamic point of view.

Stage two is the Post-MSc Training leading to a qualification as a Forensic Psychodynamic Therapist with the FPS and through this registration with the Forensic Psychodynamic Section of the BPC.

## Training course

There are three main components of the stage two training:

### *Academic teaching*

Each trainee must have completed at least 200 h of academic teaching including seminars, workshops and clinical presentations, prior to starting the training. In most cases this will have been by completing step 1 training – (i.e. the MSc in Psychotherapeutic Approaches in Mental Health and Forensic Settings). This is built on further by regular academic seminars on at least a monthly basis during the training period until qualification (a minimum of two years). Seminars are also made available through tele-conferencing facilities to facilitate long-distance learning and training.

Psychoanalytic theory prior to and during training is taught by experienced and knowledgeable practitioners and encompasses a thorough grounding in theory and psychoanalytic thought, using the current, extensive, published literature. A wide range of psychoanalytic approaches is also taught, including those directly relevant to the forensic setting (individual and organisational), to enable trainees to develop a flexible but thorough understanding of the theory base and to encourage critical appraisal of theory.

Clinical presentations expose the trainees to different clinical approaches in the field from those offered by their supervisors and training therapists. In clinical seminars, trainees take turns to present their clinical work to the seminar leader and other trainees in conditions of strict confidentiality.

### *Supervision*

Prior to starting training each candidate will usually have completed at least six terms of weekly supervision in application groups in which they present clinical material as a component of the MSc in Psychotherapeutic Approaches (or equivalent). Whilst in training, each trainee treats a minimum of two Forensic Psychotherapy Training patients, for a minimum of one year each. The patients should be one of each sex, and treated a minimum of once weekly. Trainees are supervised weekly, for about one hour each time, normally by an experienced BPC registered psychoanalytic psychotherapist with experience working in forensic settings, on an individual or small group (maximum of three participant students) basis, and have a different supervisor for each case – again, usually one of each sex. This supervision continues until qualification.

All cases must be assessed by the FPS Training Committee as suitable cases for treatment by a trainee under careful supervision. The training adheres to the BPC's protocol for clinical responsibility for training cases.

The supervision consists of a detailed discussion of the clinical material presented by the trainee about the treatment sessions. The trainee is required to bring comprehensive notes detailing the interactions and dialogue of the treatment session; the supervisor will be informed of all the details about the patient in order to safeguard the treatment and the patient's best interests.

Supervisors are selected by the FPS Training Committee, which has clear written criteria and procedures in place. However, normally supervisors should be BPC registrants, with five years' post-qualification experience of both intensive and non-intensive psychoanalytic psychotherapy with adults in forensic settings.

### *Personal psychoanalytic psychotherapy (training therapy)*

Prior to training, the candidate will have participated in 30 weekly Experiential Groups conducted by a BPC registrant or equivalent. Whilst in training trainees must have personal psychoanalytic psychotherapy for at least six months before starting their academic seminars and continue for the duration of the training – i.e. until qualification. Frequency of personal therapy must be of the same frequency as the training cases that are seen by the student as a minimum requirement (i.e. if the personal therapy is once weekly the cases can only be once weekly); however, three times weekly work would be encouraged if possible.

Normally training therapists are BPC clinical practitioner registrants (psychoanalytic psychotherapy/psychoanalysis/Jungian analysis category) with five years' post-qualification experience of both intensive and non-intensive psychoanalytic psychotherapy with adults.

## Assessment of trainees

Trainees should be involved in workplace-based assessment throughout their training and given written feedback at least once per year. The assessment should include feedback from all relevant staff involved with the trainee with the exception of the training therapist. The trainees' regular reports on their patients, and their contribution to theoretical and clinical seminars should be discussed and critically evaluated by the staff who know the trainee well. Also experienced colleagues should be involved who do not know the trainee well but can provide a more distanced assessment of the clinical standard of the trainee as shown in their clinical reports and their clinical discussions in seminars.

In the appointment of training therapists and supervisors, if the FPS Training Committee considers, in exceptional circumstances, that there is a suitable applicant who does not meet the stated criteria, they have discretion to look at the individual concerned and appoint them according to their own equivalency criteria. However, this will only be in exceptional circumstances. Normally heads of training, and senior staff members, should be BPC registrants and eligible to be training therapists and supervisors.

## The Forensic Psychotherapy Society

The result of all these recent efforts is the birth of a new Member Institution of the BPC, the FPS, which provides both a framework for a national training and multidisciplinary professional pathway in psychodynamic forensic psychotherapy and also the potential future development of an active post-qualification organisation supporting CPD and all other forms of professional development. Jessica Yakeley and Celia Taylor were particularly helpful in encouraging a collaborative working relationship between the new Society and the International Association of Forensic Psychotherapy. The Forensic Psychotherapy Section of the Association of Psychoanalytic Psychotherapy in the NHS has also contributed to this innovative project. The ultimate common aim is to realise the objective, stated throughout this paper, of establishing a critical mass of skilled professionals who can contribute to a cultural change in our forensic institutions, in the penal system and in probation services.

## Disclosure statement

No potential conflict of interest was reported by the authors.

## References

Fallon, P., Bluglass, R., Edwards, B., & Daniels, G. (1999). *Report of the committee of inquiry into the personality disorder unit*. Ashworth Special Hospital. Retrieved from http://www.gov.uk

Hollway, W. (2001). The psycho-social subject in 'evidence-based practice'. *Journal of Social Work Practice, 15*, 9–22.

Kirtchuk, G., Gordon, J., McAlister, M., & Reiss, D. (2013). *Interpersonal dynamics consultation: A manual for clinicians*. London: The Forensic Education Department and the Forensic Psychotherapy Department, West London Mental Health NHS Trust.

Reiss, D., & Kirtchuk. G. (n.d.). E-learning app. A free iPhone and iPad application on interpersonal dynamics available from the Apple store.

Reiss, D., & Kirtchuk, G. (2009). Interpersonal dynamics and multidisciplinary teamwork. *Advances in Psychiatric Treatment, 15*, 462–469.

# Index

Note: Page numbers followed by 'n' refer to notes
Page numbers in **bold** refer to figures

# INDEX

For Product Safety Concerns and Information please contact our EU
representative GPSR@taylorandfrancis.com
Taylor & Francis Verlag GmbH, Kaufingerstraße 24, 80331 München, Germany

www.ingramcontent.com/pod-product-compliance
Ingram Content Group UK Ltd.
Pitfield, Milton Keynes, MK11 3LW, UK
UKHW011011180926
475701UK00004B/688

* 9 7 8 0 3 6 7 2 2 9 6 1 0 *